LISTENING
WITH LOVE

PASTORAL COUNSELLING
A CHRISTIAN RESPONSE TO PEOPLE LIVING WITH HIV/AIDS

LISTENING
WITH LOVE

PASTORAL COUNSELLING
A CHRISTIAN RESPONSE TO PEOPLE LIVING WITH HIV/AIDS

Fr Robert Igo OSB

World Council of Churches, Geneva

Edited by Jack Messenger
Design and layout: Keith Shaw, Threefold Design Ltd
Cover photo: Small girl in village near Zimmi, Sierra Leone.
Peter Williams, WCC

ISBN: 2-8254-1454-9

Website: http://www.wcc-coe.org

Printed in France

Contents

Preface

The ecumenical movement has been highlighting the HIV and AIDS issue since the 1980s. In 1986 the World Council of Churches recommended three main areas for the churches' response: pastoral care, social ministry and education/prevention. Since then, the WCC has launched a variety of initiatives and developed and distributed various publications to assist churches in overcoming the pandemic. *The Guide to HIV and AIDS Pastoral Counselling*, published in 1990, was a significant step and has been greatly appreciated and widely utilized.

During the past 15 years, the HIV and AIDS pandemic has spread far and wide, affecting regions across the world. Throughout this period, congregations and Christian communities have been at the forefront, facing the pandemic on their own doorsteps and responding with care and support. The pandemic has mobilized Christian communities worldwide. But this enthusiasm and commitment is not yet universal and needs to become the norm. Communities are willing to bring about a tangible and positive difference in people's lives; they need to be better equipped to do so.

Listening with Love is designed as a Bible-based resource book to assist congregations in effective pastoral counselling in a time of HIV and AIDS. It is an attempt to "open the floodgates of heaven" (2 Kings 7:2): to resist the siege that communities experience due to the barriers with which humankind divides itself in the form of ignorance, poverty and stigmatization; to let the grace of God flow freely into all our lives; to unleash the healing power of God among people; to assist us to accompany, care and serve. For it is by listening that we receive God. It is by serving others that we see God. It is by empowering those who are living with HIV and AIDS that communities will be liberated from the pandemic. May God bless us all in this endeavour.

Dr Manoj Kurian
Programme executive
Health and Healing
World Council of Churches

Introduction

This manual is a Christian response to HIV/AIDS. Before you read any further, why not stop for a moment to reflect and pray?

Read John 20:11–18
What thoughts come into your mind as you read this passage?
Are there any links between it and the HIV/AIDS pandemic?
Has it anything to say about the way we approach a Christian ministry of listening?

There are many millions of women, men, young people and children throughout the world who are weeping because of the devastation of HIV and AIDS. Like Mary, they are looking for hope and sometimes, like her, they look for this hope in the wrong place and in the wrong way.

Mary went into the garden looking for the wrong thing. She went to look for a dead body, and she encountered the risen Jesus. She wanted to do things for him: 'Tell me where you've put him and I will …' A woman alone picking up a dead body – is that reasonable?

If we desire to listen with love to those who are infected with and affected by HIV/AIDS we need to be clear what kind of service we hope to provide. Perhaps our ideas may need to change so that we too encounter the risen Jesus in the very people we want to accompany. Pastoral counselling of those infected with HIV and AIDS is primarily about finding life and being life giving. As Christians who are inspired by the gospel of life we can be a genuine source of compassion, healing and encouragement through a ministry of listening love.

Let's pray:

Lord Jesus, I trust in you.

My desire is to be a living expression of your compassion and care. In your ministry you listened to those in pain and tried to bring to them healing and peace. Send now the gift of your Holy Spirit to anoint my ears and heart so that I too can learn how to listen to the cries of your people and that through a ministry of listening love I may bring to those who are most in need of you an awareness of your healing presence. Amen.

Basic questions

This introduction answers three basic questions:

* Why is this manual necessary?
* What does it contain?
* How can it be used?

AIDS has been with us for more than 20 years. It will continue to challenge us for many decades to come. The most important lesson we have learnt so far is that we can make a difference: we can prevent new infections, we can improve the quality of care and treatment for people living with HIV.

Kofi Annan, UN Secretary General, *2004 Report on the Global AIDS Epidemic*

If you are reading this manual you are probably already interested and involved in the care or counselling of those living with HIV/AIDS. You will know from first-hand experience how demanding caring for others can be. Perhaps you've opened this manual in the hope of finding encouragement or simply to be informed. Whatever the reason, you will certainly want to be more effective in bringing hope and compassion.

When God went into the garden to see Adam and Eve he did so in order to listen to their story. At the heart of the Christian faith is a ministry of listening, which allows people to come out of hiding and to tell their own story in their own way, so as to find meaning, hope and direction.

It is this ministry of compassionate listening and care that is one of the greatest contributions that we as Christians can offer in the face of the HIV/AIDS pandemic. What follows is a small attempt to encourage this Christian ministry, so that we can journey confidently with those who are infected with and affected by the virus and begin together to create communities of healing and life.

Creating 'safe spaces' for telling one's own story within our church communities is therefore a practical step through which congregations can become healing communities. The church, which is built upon and shaped around the master story of the gospels, can offer a forum where those who are afflicted can, in trust and acceptance, let down their guards and share their stories.

WCC, *Facing AIDS*

Why is this manual necessary?

It is currently estimated that 38 million people worldwide are living with the HIV/AIDS virus. It is the most serious health crisis of modern times. Women, men and children of all ages, irrespective of their education, social status and religious beliefs, are struggling. We cannot ignore them.

The battle against AIDS ought to be everyone's battle.

Pope John Paul II

We have to make people everywhere understand that the AIDS crisis is not over; that this is not about a few foreign countries, far away. This is a threat to an entire generation; this is a threat to our civilization.

Kofi Annan, UN Secretary General: Special Assembly on HIV/AIDS, June 2001

We know that HIV/AIDS strikes at every level of life. It goes to the heart of what it means to be human, and it raises issues of economic stability, gender inequality, justice and spirituality. Fear and ignorance about the nature of this virus, as well as confused understandings about our sexuality and the place of God in the struggle with HIV/AIDS, must not prevent us from promoting a genuine pastoral approach.

Through baptism, people of faith are called to share in the ministry of Jesus. We are invited to establish healing communities in the midst of pain and suffering, whatever their nature or source. Christians have been asked to console (2 Corinthians 1:3–5), to reconcile (2 Corinthians 5:19), to love (1 Corinthians 13) and to be with and serve others (Matthew 25:35–36). Throughout history those who have encountered Jesus Christ in their own lives have committed themselves to serve others, especially the poor, the sick, the destitute and the dying. We are challenged to see Christ in the poorest of the poor, no matter how their poverty manifests itself.

This manual seeks to promote the gospel of compassion. It is based on a hunger for hope and life. As people committed to life in all its fullness (John 10:10) we wish to help all people to discover God in their lives. Our belief encourages us to accompany those living with HIV/AIDS and join them in breaking down barriers of stigma and discrimination, ignorance and fear. We want to provide pastoral support so that their concerns and worries, needs and desires may find an appropriate and informed structure of care and counselling.

> Pastoral care is a sign of Jesus' presence. It gives good news to the suffering. The pastoral caregiver must be a messenger of Christ's hope and healing.
>
> John Muchiri, *HIV/AIDS: Breaking the Silence*

What will you find in this manual?

This manual will help you feel comfortable and confident in listening to people living with HIV/AIDS. It will provide you with some basic skills so that you can help other people express their pain, suffering and confusion, their anger, doubts and fears, in a safe and healing environment. It will not train you to become a professional counsellor, but it will help you improve your counselling skills so that you can listen more effectively and professionally.

The manual presents a Christian understanding of care and counselling in the context of HIV/AIDS. It will help you to help others help themselves. Christian caregivers try to empower those infected and affected, so that they may find within themselves the sources of healing and strength that are God's gifts.

Read John 7:37–40

If anyone is thirsty, let them come to me and drink. Whoever believes in me, as scripture has said, streams of living water will flow from within them.

1 Corinthians 3:16–17; 6:19–20

Do you not know that you are the temple of the Holy Spirit?

Revelation 22:1–6

On each side of the river stood the tree of life bearing twelve crops of fruit, yielding its fruit each month. And the leaves of the trees are for healing of the nations.

Faced with a life-threatening disease, people begin to ask questions:

* Where is God to be found in this virus and in this suffering?
* What is my value as a human being?
* What is the purpose of life and death?
* How may I forgive or be forgiven?
* How can I live without giving up hope?

Pastoral counselling needs to be organized and life-affirming if it is to help people answer such questions. We need to be a listening, loving presence in our communities. This manual will provide you with structure and direction so that you can listen more effectively to those living with HIV/AIDS. It is not the final word on the subject, but it is a resource that you can adapt to your own situation and cultural setting.

How can this manual be used?

In hospitals, clinics, home-based care of the sick and dying, the conducting of funerals and through prayer and worship, many Christians (and other faith-based groups) are involved in pastoral support for people living with HIV/AIDS.

This manual will provide you with confidence and encouragement. It challenges others to consider offering themselves in the service of their brothers and sisters through a ministry of listening with love. It is an attempt to help us all feel more comfortable with the invitation to listen to those living with HIV/AIDS, so that we can help them in their daily struggle to find a way of living positively.

1   It will inform all of us about the physical and spiritual concerns surrounding HIV/AIDS. Having the right information helps dispel confusion and ignorance.
2   Christian groups who wish to take seriously the call to fight stigma and discrimination can use this manual as a starting point for discussion. They can then devise their own appropriate and focused compassionate response, based on the actual needs and resources of their locality.
3   Individuals may use this manual to equip themselves with the skills that will best contribute to providing a safe place for others to share their stories.

It will be important to reflect as you read and to adapt what you learn to your own needs and circumstances. No one can tell us *exactly* how to care and counsel others, for each situation is different and we need to learn to respond to and respect the person before us. However, we can support each other by sharing our experience. This manual offers such support.

One thing we can be sure of is that we have what it takes to fight this pandemic because we have all it takes to conquer – **we have Christ!**

Sr Tarisai Zata OP, Dominican Sister in Zimbabwe

Let's Begin at the Beginning

This chapter answers the following questions:

* What is HIV/AIDS?
* What does it mean to be HIV-positive?
* How do I know whether I am HIV-positive?
* How does the HIV virus progress into AIDS?
* What are the main routes of HIV transmission?
* Who is at risk and how can risk be avoided?

It is now common knowledge that in HIV/AIDS, it is not the condition itself that hurts most (because many other diseases and conditions lead to serious suffering and death), but the stigma and the possibility of rejection and discrimination, misunderstanding and loss of trust that HIV-positive people have to deal with.

Canon Gidean Byamugisha, *WCC, Plan of Action*

Ignorance is still a major factor in the spread of HIV/AIDS, even after 22 years of information. If we wish to provide an effective pastoral ministry of listening and care then we need to make sure that we are properly informed about HIV and AIDS, otherwise we will only pass on our own ignorance and fear.

What is HIV/AIDS?

Before reading any further, ask yourself:

* What do I already know about HIV/AIDS?
* How would I explain the difference between HIV and AIDS?
* Am I clear about how the virus is transmitted?
* Where am I lacking in knowledge?

Since the early 1980s we have known about the existence of a disease called AIDS. Many people know that AIDS stands for Acquired Immune Deficiency Syndrome.

We also know that a virus called HIV causes AIDS. HIV stands for Human Immunodeficiency Virus.

HIV attacks a person's immune system and makes them less able to fight sickness. The person usually goes on to develop the disease called AIDS, a disease that is at present incurable. It is important to remember that a person who is infected by HIV does not develop the symptoms either of the virus or the disease called AIDS straight away. That is why you cannot tell whether or not a person has HIV or AIDS simply by looking at them. It can take two to ten years after infection before any signs of illness begin to show. Once infected, however, a person remains infected for life and can infect others.

HIV and AIDS are primarily medical conditions, but they cause many other distressing problems. Thus, we must not limit ourselves to medical information alone. And as we shall see, HIV may cause AIDS, but the risks of HIV infection depend on many different factors.

What does it mean to be HIV-positive?

For a disease to take root in us it needs to attach itself somehow or enter the cells of the body. HIV attacks a type of white blood cell called the T-helper cell. It does this by breaking down a door in the cell called the CD4-receptor. Once inside, the HIV virus disguises itself so that it is hard to detect, and then multiplies.

Having fooled the body's natural immune system the HIV virus then puts it out of action. Once this has been achieved (or the immune system is at least severely weakened) other diseases can take advantage and attack the body. We call such diseases opportunistic infections.

Thus we see why HIV is so dangerous: it disables the very system that should protect us. The body's natural 'burglar alarm' is turned off and it is too late to defend ourselves. HIV is so clever that it can disguise itself to look like the very cell it attacks. By the time it has been unmasked, the immune system has been destroyed.

She had been married for seven years and had been subjected to physical abuse constantly. Her husband used to beat her over trivial issues. For example, one time he beat her because he accused her of being rude to a neighbour. During one of the beatings her husband told her that he had infected her with AIDS. After this she went for a test and she was found to be HIV-positive.

Following another beating she was admitted to hospital for suspected meningitis, but it was later discovered that during the beatings she had sustained head injuries. After leaving the hospital the beatings got worse and so she went to the police and talked to her relatives, but nothing happened. She felt that she could not go on with the marriage.

She then spoke to a pastoral counsellor from her church. Together, they looked at her options: staying at a shelter for survivors of domestic violence, going to court and getting her share of the property, joining a support group for women with HIV, having further counselling. She decided to pursue all the options, as she wanted to live positively with HIV but free from violence.

South African AIDS Training Programme, May 2001

Yet living with HIV and AIDS means much more than having to suffer from infections. We also live with fear: fear of telling others because of what they may think or say, fear of death and how difficult it might be, fear of the future and what this will mean for our partner, spouse or children.

We also live with the anger at how this virus first came into our bodies. Often, we live with the need to forgive: to forgive ourselves, as well as others. Depending on where we are in the world, we may have to cope with the pressure of trying to find enough money for medication and food. We live with the questions: 'How can I learn to live with a virus that would like to kill me? How can this enemy become a friend?'

To be HIV-positive and to live with AIDS means we are infected on every level of our lives: physical, psychological, spiritual, social and economic. HIV and AIDS make us question our lifestyles. Why should this virus have entered our lives in the first place? What kind of God would allow this to happen? We face many spiritual questions once we are diagnosed. Our faith in God and our self-worth take a real battering.

How do I know whether I am HIV-positive?

The only sure way to know our status is to have an HIV antibody test. It is important to understand exactly what an HIV test is and what it is not.

An HIV test does not reveal whether someone has AIDS. Rather, it detects the antibodies that attack the body's immune system. Antibodies are substances produced by the white blood cells. Most people will produce antibodies if the HIV virus infects them, though not straight away. There is always a gap between being infected and the appearance of the antibodies in the blood. This is often referred to as the window period. However, within a relatively short time a person who has been infected will develop a level of antibodies that can be detected.

If a person is concerned about their HIV status then it is best for them to be tested as soon as possible after the time when they think they could have been exposed. Once a person decides to go for a test the procedure is simple. Different testing agencies have different practices, but the basic steps are as follows:

* The person is asked why they would like to be tested and what their knowledge of HIV/AIDS is.
* A laboratory technician or nurse takes a sample of blood.
* If the test is a 'rapid test' they may wait for the results. Otherwise, a further appointment is made.
* Before the results are given the person tested meets with a counsellor in order to check what they understand by a positive or negative result and what changes they will make to their lifestyle.

Simon is 23 years old, and has just finished university. Recently, he went to a clinic for a minor health problem and had the following conversation with the doctor in charge: 'I can treat you, Simon', the doctor said to him, 'but we need to talk a little more about your sickness.'

Simon immediately became anxious and asked if this was unusual. The doctor told him that it looked like a sexually transmitted disease. When he heard this, he immediately began sweating and mentioning a relationship that he had had previously.

'Simon, I can see you are afraid', the doctor said. 'Some laboratory tests need to be done so that we can determine exactly what you are suffering from.'

The doctor explained about the tests, including the HIV test, and made sure that he understood why it was important to know his status. The HIV test was positive. The doctor counselled Simon and encouraged him to see a pastoral counsellor at his local church, for he knew Simon was a Christian.

'No!' Simon yelled back at the doctor. 'I cannot be HIV-positive, and I won't go to any pastoral counsellor!'

He left feeling very angry and full of anxiety. He thought of death, and felt rejected. He even thought about suicide. He was depressed and felt hopeless. He remained like this for months without telling anyone. He went to work and tried to act as if nothing was wrong. If anyone found out, he thought that would be the end, he would lose his job.

After about six months life got so difficult that in the end he told a friend about his HIV status. Though he felt relieved he soon became more concerned once he realized that his friend had betrayed his confidence. Finally, desperation drove him to go to the pastoral counsellor at his church.

John Muchiri, *HIV/AIDS: Breaking the Silence*

How does the HIV virus progress into AIDS?

There are four basic stages once a person has been infected.

STAGE 1 A person is infected with HIV

At first, a person does not look sick, nor do they feel unwell. It is not possible to decide whether or not they are HIV-positive simply by looking at them. After some time, however, they may find that they are getting frequent bouts of tiredness, fevers, aching muscles, colds and flu's, and other infections. Remember: even though people look and feel healthy, they can still be infected.

STAGE 2 They develop symptoms related to AIDS

As a person's immune system becomes weaker they may develop symptoms related to AIDS. They experience loss of weight, loss of appetite, sores in the mouth, diarrhoea, swollen lymph glands, skin rashes, fever and night sweats. We need to be careful, however, as these can also be the symptoms of many other illnesses. If someone is concerned they should see a doctor or go for an HIV test.

STAGE 3 They develop AIDS

AIDS is a result of being infected by HIV, when the body's immune system cannot fight off serious infections. It is impossible to say exactly what disease a person may get, as these can vary depending on the environment. A person becomes ill and is then diagnosed with an AIDS related illness. Common diseases are tuberculosis, herpes zoster, chronic diarrhoea, weight loss, intestinal infections, meningitis and certain cancers.

Stage 4 They die of an AIDS related illness

Without a functioning immune system no one can live. Medication has improved the quality of life for many who live with AIDS and has lengthened their lives. Without adequate medication, however, they will die of an AIDS related disease. This is much more likely to happen in the developing world.

What are the main routes of HIV transmission?

HIV is found mainly in the blood, semen, vaginal fluids and breast milk of infected people. In order for the virus to spread, one of these bodily fluids must pass from one person to another. Unless it has cuts or sores, our skin is thick enough to keep out HIV. The vagina and rectum, however, have a thinner covering of skin, which can easily break. This is why the virus can get into the bloodstream more easily at these points.

There are four main ways that HIV can enter the bloodstream:

* Sexual intercourse with an infected person.
* Through transfusions of contaminated blood, via unsterilized instruments, and other blood-to-blood contact.
* From an HIV-positive mother to her child in the womb.
* Breast feeding by a mother who is HIV-positive.

In the first three there must be a person who is infected, who in turn passes on the virus through blood or vaginal or seminal fluid. This often occurs through the mucous membrane of the mouth, vagina or rectum, or a break in the skin.

There are still many myths about HIV/AIDS. We know that this virus cannot be transmitted by:

* touching
* sharing the same blankets or cups and plates
* shaking hands
* living in the same house
* insect bites

Simply being in the same room as a person who is infected with HIV/AIDS cannot put us at risk. However, if we are caring for a relative or friend who is very sick with HIV/AIDS, we will of course need to take some care about soiled linen and coming into contact with blood.

TO SPEAK ONLY OF THE MEDICAL CAUSES OF HIV/AIDS IS TO NEGLECT THE MANY OTHER FACTORS THAT CONTRIBUTE TO THE SPREAD OF THIS PANDEMIC.

LACK OF LEADERSHIP   POVERTY   GENDER ISSUES

HIV AIDS

CULTURAL BELIEFS AND PRACTICES   ECONOMIC FACTORS

Who is at risk and how can risk be avoided?

From what we have discussed so far it will be clear that certain behaviours put us at risk more than others. This is especially true when we are sexually active. Risk factors include the following:

* Having sexual intercourse when you or your partner has a sexually transmitted disease.
* Having sex if there are sores or bleeding around the genital area.
* Having many sexual partners.
* Having sex with someone whose HIV status is unknown.
* Having sex without the use of a condom.
* Being injected with a contaminated needle or other equipment.
* Sharing non-sterile needles or syringes.
* Being circumcised, tattooed, engaging in blood-mixing rituals or being cut with any instrument that is not sterilized after each use.
* Coming into contact with body fluids and soiled sheets.

Read Romans 12:1–12

Risk, however, is not simply about behaviour. We can be at risk because of poverty, lack of social support, war, gender and our age. In many parts of the world women and girls are most at risk because of their biological makeup and because they are discriminated against and disadvantaged. Children, too, can be at risk via rape and sexual abuse because in some parts of the world they are thought to be free from the disease or considered to bring cleansing and healing through sexual activity.

Homosexual women and men, and intravenous drug users, likewise are at risk due to marginalization and discrimination.

After 22 years of HIV/AIDS, we now realize that this pandemic is not simply a health issue, but something that affects all aspects of human life. Where there is poverty, gender inequality, human rights violations, child abuse, racism, economic instability, or war and violence, then HIV/AIDS will thrive.

If we want to take seriously the things that contribute to the spread of HIV/AIDS, we can no longer limit ourselves to simply talking about sexual morality or the need to change individual behaviour. Rather, we need to face the fact that some people's choices have already been made for them because of the structure of society. Individuals may desire to change, but they may not have the freedom to do so. Their decisions may not be supported by the structures of society around them. Structural sin is as real as individual sin. In this sense we need to be aware that it is not simply individuals that are flawed, but structures as well.

* How would the word of God help us avoid being infected?
* In what way can we offer our bodies as a living sacrifice?
* What practical steps can we take and encourage others to take in order to remain free from infection?
* What kind of compassion are we going to have for those whose behaviour has put them at risk?

In providing pastoral care for those most at risk we must also highlight the abuses that continue to put people at risk in the first place.

The Christian Response

This chapter will answer the following questions:

* What has HIV/AIDS to do with Christians?
* Is HIV/AIDS a punishment from God for sin?
* Don't people bring HIV/AIDS upon themselves?
* So why do people suffer?
* How have Christians responded to the HIV/AIDS pandemic?

HIV and Aids is not asking anything new from the religious community, rather AIDS is confronting us with the reality of becoming more fully the kind of people we have been called to be.

Unknown source

Why should we worry about those who have HIV? Isn't it their own fault? They've brought this disease upon themselves!

Where is the forgiveness and understanding that Jesus came to bring? My husband gave me this virus. Should I now be ashamed, full of guilt?

What has HIV/AIDS to do with Christians?

Silence and denial, or pointing a finger in blame and shame, are not helpful responses to HIV/AIDS. Christians are not only affected by the pandemic; many of us are also infected. The Body of Christ is suffering from HIV/AIDS. As followers of Jesus, we have a duty to respond.

Many people claim to have no faith, and even we who believe in God and in the promises of Jesus find the existence of the HIV/AIDS pandemic a challenge. We don't find any easy answers in the person of Jesus, but we do see one who himself was unfairly labelled and discriminated against. If we examine the life of Jesus, we find someone who suffered physically and emotionally. In Jesus, we can also find healing and strength.

Read Mark 5:25–34

Because she had heard about Jesus, this woman came up behind him and touched his cloak thinking, 'If I just touch his clothing, I shall get well.' Then Jesus said to her, 'Daughter, your faith has saved you; go in peace and be free of this illness.'

Jesus' own life and ministry are full of examples of his desire to bring comfort to those in distress. He healed all diseases unconditionally (Mark 1:29–32) and reached out to those who were stigmatized (Mark 1:40–45; Luke 17:11–19). He forgave sins (John 8:1–12; Luke 7:36–49; 15:11–32), took the side of those who were poor (Matthew 9:10–13; Luke 18:1–8) and denounced oppressive social structures (Luke 4:16–22).

As Christian pastoral caregivers, we can bring hope and encouragement as we seek to bring what practical assistance we can to the difficult situations faced by individuals and families. We can bring a listening presence that gives people time and opportunity to discover for themselves where God may be found. By means of scripture and prayer, we can find hope and meaning where they seemed lost. HIV and AIDS are concerns of Christians because they are concerns of God.

Read Mark 1:29–34

The sick came to Jesus looking for consolation. Can we turn people away in our own day? Wherever there was sickness, Jesus was found bringing healing.

Read James 5:13–18

In our Christian communities there are always people who are sick or in need of pastoral support. They need our prayers and our compassionate presence. These can often provide the healing love and emotional help for which they hunger.

Is HIV/AIDS a punishment from God for sin?

The simple answer is no.

For too long in the minds of some Christians, all sickness – especially HIV and AIDS – has been regarded as the result of sin. Sickness has always puzzled people, which is perhaps why some have thought: 'If God is a God of love, then surely sickness must come as a form of punishment for our own bad actions and choices? If we are good, then we will be healthy and prosper. If we do evil then God will take away his love from us!' However, there are many examples of good people who die of cancer or other diseases, and of babies who are born with disabilities. What have they done to deserve punishment? Isn't this what the Book of Job struggles with?

HIV/AIDS has particularly been associated with a lack of morality, in a simplistic but deadly chain of consequences:

HIV = Sex = Sin = Punishment = Death

Such thinking is not to be found in the example and teaching of Jesus.

Read John 8:1–11; 9:1–5; Mark 2:1–5

As we reflect on these passages can we really think that in our own day Jesus would condemn people and want to see them suffer? The disciples asked the question 'who sinned?' but for Jesus this is not the important issue. When people are sick the most important question is not how they became sick, but what can we do to help them in their suffering.

Don't people bring HIV/AIDS upon themselves?

Jesus has taught us not to judge (John 8:15). Of course, choices have consequences. Whatever we do in life can have an effect on our health and well-being. All of us need to learn how to choose life, rather than death (Deuteronomy 30:19). Yet no one is ever totally free in the choices they make. Our culture, our economic and social environments, our beliefs and values influence our choices. As Christians, however, we are asked to be compassionate (Matthew 6). That does not mean blaming others, but standing with them in their need.

HIV has in many situations become associated purely with sexual activity, even though sex is not the only way that people can become infected. And, of course, many women and young girls become HIV-positive while remaining faithful to one partner – their husbands. Still others have little choice about whether or not to be sexually active.

Undue interest in how a person became HIV-positive is not a feature of the pastoral counsellor or caregiver. Our task is to face the suffering at hand and to bring encouragement.

Betty Strauss was diagnosed HIV-positive in November 1998, after the death of her husband. Soon she noticed that people were avoiding her and didn't want her near their children. Feeling desperate, she spoke to the pastor of the church she attended. 'I wanted to tell the congregation that I had HIV but I didn't have AIDS.' The pastor listened but would not allow her to speak in church. He never visited her at home; neither did any of the elders of the church. 'I felt that no one from the church wanted anything to do with me.'

One Saturday afternoon in September 2000, Betty noticed a march through the centre of Windhoek. People were carrying banners and posters about HIV and AIDS. It was a March for Hope for Namibia's orphans, organized by Catholic AIDS Action. One of the marchers gave Betty a leaflet, where she read about the Bernhard Nardkamp Centre, which she decided to visit. It was two weeks before she had enough money for the bus fare, but she finally saved enough money and found the place.

'I found everything I was looking for and it has been important for my life and health. We always pray together. It's important for me to pray because it helps me to look beyond this sickness. It helps me to take each day at a time and I've come to understand the suffering of human beings. I've also suffered in many ways and life has been far from easy, but I now understand that whatever happens, my life has a purpose.'

G. Williams and A. Williams, *Journeys of Faith*

So why do people suffer?

There is of course no easy answer to this question, but as Christians we must struggle to make sense of this fundamental fact of life. Whether we like it or not, or whether we understand it or not, people do suffer.

* Why do people suffer?
* Why do we bring suffering upon others and ourselves?
* Why is there disease?
* Why does God allow rape and sexual abuse of innocent children?

Faced with suffering, we begin to question the purpose and meaning of life and the things we value. We question our faith and what kind God we actually believe in. Suffering causes us to struggle with the big question of *why*?

Christianity tries to deal with the problem of suffering honestly and seriously. This is because the Christian faith has at its heart the belief in a crucified God. Paul speaks about this clearly:

The language of the cross remains nonsense for those who are lost. Yet for us who are saved, it is the power of God ... The Jews ask for miracles and the Greeks for a higher knowledge, while we preach a crucified Messiah. (1 Corinthians 1:18–23)

The Christian faith speaks of a God who not only experienced agonizing physical pain, but also the deeper wound of rejection and abandonment from those he loved and tried to help. In this sense our Christian faith does not try to run away from the presence of suffering in the world, but rather it attempts to point beyond it. The ugly face of suffering not only keeps our feet firmly rooted in the reality of life, but also clearly reminds us that there are no simple answers.

I have no clever answer to the eternal 'Why?' of suffering but I am convinced that whatever its cause and whatever its outcome, it is never without meaning. Just what that meaning is I can only guess: perhaps different people's suffering has different meanings. Some are clearly purified and strengthened by it and go on to do great things for God and his people. Others are quite simply broken, dehumanized and destroyed. Some are ruined before they can even begin: the parcel unwrapped with such eagerness and hope reveals only a pitiful collection of broken shards, wrecked beyond any hope of repair.

Sheila Cassidy, *Good Friday People*

Why people suffer is not always clear, but we do not need to lose hope. Paul in his letter to the Romans explains that 'nothing can separate us from the love of God' (Romans 8:38–39). God is not to be found outside of our suffering, but in the very centre of our struggle and pain. We cannot avoid the difficulties that we will encounter in life, but we can begin to choose how we interpret them. Suffering is a mystery. We do not know why people are raped or murdered, why there are diseases that cause death, why some people feel that suicide is the answer to their problems. It is not clever answers that will bring relief, but the knowledge that there is a power greater than ourselves who can help us through the pain and confusion.

I have long since given up asking the 'why' of suffering. It gets us nowhere … I know less and less, but that which I do know, I know ever more deeply … suffering is, in the same way that life is … more important than asking why, we should get in there, be alongside those who suffer.

Sheila Cassidy, *Good Friday People*

All of us need a reason to live and the more we come face to face with suffering the deeper this need becomes. The mystery of suffering leaves us with many unanswered questions, yet it also takes us to the heart of our faith and the heart of our God. Having been created by a God of tenderness and compassion we find our very dignity and destiny in our humanity.

How have Christians responded to the HIV/AIDS pandemic?

From the very beginning of the HIV/AIDS pandemic, Christians – along with many others – have tried to bring relief and help to those affected, including widows and orphans, the dead and the dying. Christian communities have brought medical assistance to millions of people, many of whom would not otherwise have received it. Through schools and youth organizations they have spread the message of prevention. Christian ministers and lay people give spiritual support to those who are dying and have conducted many funerals. Christians have also been in the forefront of advocacy and lobbying for antiretroviral drugs (which reduce the levels of HIV in the bloodstream) and adequate mother-to-child transmission programmes.

There are many other admirable examples of the gospel of compassion and self-giving. The question is not 'Have Christians done anything?' Rather, it is 'What more can be done?' Stephan Lewis, UN Special Envoy for HIV/AIDS in Africa, spoke to religious leaders gathered in Nairobi in July 2002:

Who else, beyond yourselves, is so well placed to lead? Who else has such a network of voices at the grassroots level? Who else has access to all communities once a week, every week, across the continent? Who else officiates at millions of funerals of those who die of AIDS related illnesses, and better understands the consequences for children and families? Who else works on a daily basis with faith-based, community-based organizations? In the midst of this wanton, ravaging pandemic, it is truly like an act of divine intervention that you should be physically present everywhere, all the time. I ask you again: who else, therefore, is so well placed to lead?

How can we best provide a new form of leadership in the fight against HIV/AIDS?

Called to Care

This chapter will answer the following questions:

* How else could we care?
* How practical is our care to be?
* What pastoral care can Christians give to those living with HIV/AIDS?
* What is pastoral counselling?
* How can pastoral counselling help?
* Who does pastoral counselling?
* What are the qualities that are needed?
* Do pastoral counsellors have their own opinions?
* How can I best use myself in pastoral counselling?
* How can I help myself as a pastoral counsellor?
* How can listening to myself help others?

You cannot catch AIDS from hugging or kissing or holding hands. We are normal. We are human beings. We walk. We can talk.

Nkosi Johnson, 11-year-old boy who died of HIV/AIDS

How else could we care?

Christian communities exist because each member has in some small way experienced the healing love of God. The ministry of Jesus allowed others to find God in the circumstances of their everyday lives.

The gospel of life which Jesus brought is summed up in the teaching he gave at Nazareth (Luke 4:16–19). He came to set prisoners free, to give sight to the blind and to heal all our disease. It is this ministry of liberation that Christians continue to exercise in their communities of faith. By means of their compassion they show that no one is outside the love of God.

The church by its very nature as the Body of Christ calls its members to become healing communities. Despite the extent and complexity of the problems raised by HIV/AIDS, the churches can make an affective healing witness towards those affected.

WCC, *Facing AIDS*

To be a Christian is to share in the mission of Jesus and that means to bring good news, especially to those in greatest need. 'What do you think?' says Jesus in Matthew 18:12–14. 'If a man has a hundred sheep, and one of them has gone astray, does he not leave the 99 on the mountains and go in search … So it is not the will of my Father who is in heaven that one of these little ones should perish.'

Here is the clearest possible indication of the immense value of each individual person in the sight of God. Indeed, if we look closely at Jesus' parables and miracles, we see just how often the unimportant and insignificant, the outcast, the outsider, the stigmatized and discriminated against, are the very people with whom he chooses to associate, by healing them or sharing a meal with them. He listens to the cry of the blind beggar (Mark 10:46–52). He touches lepers and eats with tax collectors, prostitutes and Pharisees (Luke 19:1–10; Mark 5:25–33; Luke 7:37–38). Jesus' knowledge of who was acceptable to God did not always fit in with the beliefs of his contemporaries.

How practical is our care to be?

Jesus' care for others was immensely practical. The example he gives us is the basis of what we call pastoral care. In pastoral care we desire to be the hands and feet and heart of Jesus. For Christians, such care is not an optional extra, but a practical living out of the gospel of life. If we feed the hungry, visit the sick and imprisoned, and clothe the naked then we are showing kindness to Jesus himself (Matthew 25:31–46). And if one part of the body is hurting then the pain is felt throughout the body, as Paul teaches us (1 Corinthians 12:12–31; Romans 12:4–21).

We are linked together in our sorrows and joys as children of God. As a result, we alleviate the pain in others as a natural expression of our compassion and sense of belonging.

Freedom is indivisible, the chains on any one of my people are the chain on all … It was during my long lonely years in prison that my hunger for freedom of my own people became a hunger for the freedom of all people, white and black. I knew as well as I knew anything that the oppressor must be liberated just as surely as the oppressed. A man who takes another man's freedom is a prisoner of hatred; he is locked behind the bars of prejudice and narrow mindedness. I am not truly free if I am taking away someone else's freedom, just as surely as I am not free when my freedom is taken away … To be free is not merely to cast off one's chains but to live in a way that respects and enhances the freedom of others.

Nelson Mandela, *A Long Walk To Freedom*

What pastoral care can Christians give to those living with HIV/AIDS?

If the Christian church is to respond more deeply to our brothers and sisters living with HIV/AIDS it has first to learn how to listen to those who are suffering. Pastoral care is never built on a desire simply to 'do things for others', let alone to do things 'to' them. Pastoral care is built upon the important recognition that we are called as Christians to stand with others in their pain and suffering and to learn from them. We should never imagine that we have all the answers. Genuine pastoral care is ultimately concerned with being present to others, long before it is about making them objects of our charity or for us to try and 'fix' them.

As Christians who care in a pastoral context we can prepare ourselves:

* Be informed about HIV and AIDS. We should know the basic facts and not speak from ignorance. Fear can only be conquered by truth. Knowing the truth will set us free and will save lives.

Read John 8:31–32

Jesus told those Jews who believed in him: 'If you remain in my word, you will truly be my disciples, and you will know the truth, and the truth will set you free.'

* Talk openly about HIV/AIDS. We can look for occasions to discuss things with others. Talking breaks the silence of stigma and discrimination and allows faith to come to light. It provides an opportunity to highlight how the gospel of life brings hope and challenge. In our families, among our relatives, in our church meetings and worship, we can make HIV/AIDS a normal part of our conversation, teaching and preaching.

Read Mark 5:1–19

As he was getting into the boat, the man who had been possessed pleaded to remain with Jesus. But Jesus told him instead: 'Go home to your family and announce to them all that the Lord in his pity has done for you.'

* We can familiarize ourselves about our local situation. We need to be clear what the needs are in our locality. We can discover what others are doing for people living with HIV/AIDS, for people at risk, for orphans and families that are affected. We can offer our help and begin as Christian groups to fill any gaps.

Read John 6:1–13

Eight months' wages would not buy enough bread for each to have a bite! Here is a boy with five loaves and two small fish, but what is that among so many?'

* Provide support for the infected and affected. We can give support and encourage others to do the same in our church families. This can be done by either funding medical aid or through practical home-based care projects. Visiting those who are sick in their homes and hospitals and providing practical support to their families where necessary are important ways of showing focused compassion. In developing countries where poverty is a contributing factor in HIV/AIDS, we can look for ways of helping with food, cleaning and simple nursing tasks.

Read Romans 12:4–16

Let love be sincere ... hold on to what is good; love one another with mutual affection; anticipate one another in showing honour.

* Give a voice to those who have no voice. The spread of HIV/AIDS is not only a medical issue. There are social and economic factors that contribute greatly to the increase in infection. Advocacy is an important way in which Christians can contribute to the fight against this pandemic. We can raise awareness and debate about poverty, gender, cultural practices, stigma and discrimination. We can help make a difference by making public the social evils that continue to feed new infections.

Read Amos 2:6–8; 8:1–7

They sell them just for money and the needy for a pair of sandals; they tread on the head of the poor and trample them upon the dust of the earth, while they silence the right of the afflicted.

✳ We can care for the caregivers as well as the infected. When someone is sick, the focus of care and much of the energy goes towards the person who is ill, yet caregivers are also affected. They fight with fear and disappointment, anger and the need to forgive, frustration and the pain of letting go. Many emotional, physical and spiritual needs come to the surface. All caregivers, whether they are professionals or family and volunteers, need to be supported and encouraged, and allowed to rest and recuperate.

Read Matthew 11:28–30

Come to me all of you who work hard and who carry heavy burdens and I will refresh you. Take my yoke upon you and learn from me, for I am gentle and humble of heart; and you will find rest. For my yoke is good and my burden light.

These are among the very practical ways that Christian groups can contribute in a focused compassionate way to the relief of some of the suffering that surrounds HIV/AIDS. Of course, our specific localities will determine what practical and imaginative response we can make. No matter where we are, however, we can also provide desperately needed spiritual and emotional care and support.

By gathering together volunteers who are willing to visit and to listen, we give those living with HIV/AIDS the invaluable opportunity to share their worries and concerns. It is sometimes easier to do something practical (e.g. clean, go shopping or provide medication) than it is to listen with love to inner pains and frustrations for which we have no quick or ready solutions. This is why Christian churches need to think more about how we can provide genuine spiritual and emotional care through pastoral care and counselling.

What is pastoral counselling?

Within the context of pastoral care there is the specific ministry of *listening*, or what we call pastoral counselling. The HIV/AIDS pandemic challenges faith-based communities to be bearers of love and hope to those affected by the virus. We do this in practical ways by demonstrating our genuine care and concern, but also by providing opportunities for people to express and to explore the thoughts and feelings that the disease arouses within them.

Pastoral counselling
* Provides a safe place to talk and to listen.
* Helps people explore important issues that concern them.
* Does not seek to judge others.
* Looks at problems through the eyes of faith.
* Respects other people's beliefs, yet offers a challenge.
* Listens with love to be a healing presence.

Many of us have experienced the relief that comes from being able to talk to someone who has the time and willingness to listen. Pastoral counselling is a way of giving people the time and opportunity to share the deeper emotional and spiritual difficulties that they experience as people living with HIV/AIDS. These encounters are not conversations that occur simply by accident (though that may happen as well). Rather, Christian communities have learnt from experience that there is a real need to provide occasions when a more 'formal sharing' can take place. For this reason many feel the need to learn some basic skills in counselling so that they can be truly present to others and listen with greater effectiveness.

Let us look a little more closely at what counselling is. Counselling is a conversation that has a purpose and is aimed at offering support to people so as to bring about healing and personal growth. This healing and growth begins to take place when a climate of trust and acceptance is created and the person is assisted to explore and understand how to cope more effectively with life and its difficulties.

People are said to be involved in counselling when they offer time to listen to the concerns of another. Such listening provides an opportunity to clarify what is really troubling a person and to discover how they can best move towards a more resourceful way of living. Hence, listening/counselling rests on the quality of our relationship, especially the qualities of honesty, trust and confidentiality. Counselling invites us, through a caring relationship and within agreed boundaries, to provide a space for those in need to talk about what is of greatest concern to them.

Pastoral counselling is a helping relationship of care, compassion and concern that provides an opportunity for issues of faith and spirituality to surface. We seek to offer support to others by entering into their world for a short time and by our listening presence we slowly begin to see life through their eyes as they begin to express what is deep inside them. As we grow in our understanding through attentive listening we can, by means of sensitive questions and comments, help them find fresh meaning and see their difficulties in a new light.

When my husband began to get ill, I was concerned to let my children be with him. I didn't know what to say to them. I asked to talk to a pastoral counsellor from my church. We shared a lot and with her help I realized that they knew a lot already. When I was brave enough to talk to them about their father's illness they shocked me by just how much they had seen and knew. Now we can talk together, even with my husband. He loves to have my youngest child playing in his room where he is, and she loves to be there. Maybe I was more frightened than the children.

South African AIDS training programme

Our motive in pastoral counselling, for standing with others in their pain and being present to them as they express their concerns, comes from our faith in Christ. We move in this way easily between basic human issues of fear, anxiety and practical problems, to theological and spiritual explorations of where God is to be found, how to pray and where to focus on hope. In pastoral counselling, therefore, we are not doing something *to* others or even *for* them.

Instead, we are simply walking with others on their journey, as Jesus did with his disciples on the road to Emmaus (Luke 24:13–35). In chapter 4 we will explore the story of Jesus' journey to Emmaus in more detail to find a model for listening with love.

※ Pastoral counselling is a relationship of love and compassion.
※ It is not a question of someone who is superior helping someone who is weak; rather, it is a way of creating a partnership of trust and equality so that together we begin to make sense of difficulties and find healing.
※ It is a ministry that is not reserved for priests or pastors, sisters or brothers in religious life, but one that all Christians should consider.
※ In pastoral counselling we make ourselves available to others, to be present to them.

How can pastoral counselling help?

To be free and to be able to tell someone what is causing us anxiety and concern is clearly beneficial. The person who is infected with HIV/AIDS and the relatives of those who are infected are not always sure to whom they can talk. Stigma and discrimination are still very powerful factors that prevent people coming out into the open. Often, a caregiver, whether it is a nurse, volunteer or relative, has many other demands on their time and so has little opportunity to look beyond the immediate physical problems. Yet HIV/AIDS often brings fear, guilt, shame and worry about the future, as well as the need to heal the past. Such wounds are painful – no less painful than the bodily discomfort of herpes, diarrhoea or many of the other ailments that may come our way if we are infected with HIV.

These inner wounds are not visible and cannot be soothed by pills or ointments. They require the patience of someone who will let us speak about all that is deep inside. That is why pastoral counselling can help: it can give people something that is free and life giving. It can provide people with *time*.

Jesus said: 'It's not what goes into a person that makes that person unclean, but what comes out of a person' (Matthew 15:10–11). 'The mouth speaks of what fills the heart' (Matthew 12:34). In the same way, healing takes place from within. Pastoral counselling is such a source of healing. It can bring a sense of inner peace.

Pastoral counselling, therefore, is not:
* Telling others what to do
* Giving advice to people
* Giving our own opinions
* Making decisions for others

All these things prevent a person from exploring their own thoughts and feelings and finding a solution to their problems for themselves. Strange as it may sound, even sympathy is not an appropriate response. People do not need us to be sorry for them. They require us to stand with them and listen as they try to reveal what is deep within them.

The person affected by HIV/AIDS requires respect and acceptance, trust and genuine compassion. They will then be able to tell their own story in all its richness and all its poverty. Anything that prevents this story being told or puts words and interpretations into the storyteller's mouth, anything that does not belong to them, blocks the counselling process.

Pastoral counselling allows a story to unfold at its own pace and in its own way. We try to allow others to experience healing and growth by helping them explore what is difficult in their life. We try to apply insights from scripture and spirituality, psychology and common sense, *sensitively*. And we hope that these insights will lead the person to a fuller understanding, wholeness and liberation.

Who does pastoral counselling?

Pastoral counselling is not a task only undertaken by pastors, ministers or priests. All Christians can provide this important service in formal or informal settings. The most affective counsellors will of course be those who themselves live with HIV/AIDS, as they will know from their own experience the issues and problems that people most commonly encounter.

We do not have to be professionally trained, but we will certainly benefit from being skilled. If we know how to 'listen actively' with love, then we will enable others to experience the healing that comes from being listened to properly, with genuine attention. Our listening will empower them to tell their story and find their own meaning.

The pastoral counsellor is therefore:
* Someone who is willing to offer time and opportunity to others so that they can talk.
* Someone who listens to persons' concerns without judgement or attempting to give advice.
* Someone who by their sensitive use of basic counselling skills and from the perspective of faith gently guides others to a greater understanding of the problems they are experiencing.
* Someone who desires to empower others to find a new way of living.

Thus, the pastoral counsellor wants to be of service in the healing ministry of Jesus. They will discover that listening is not always easy or simple. Giving their attention to others can be demanding and requires a lot of energy. They need specific qualities within themselves to enable them to carry out their ministry of listening most effectively.

What are the qualities that are needed?

The pastoral counsellor is one who listens as someone tries to tell his or her own story. Hence, acceptance and warmth are essential qualities. There are also other important qualities that will help us listen to what is *really* being said, rather than what we *think* is being said. There are three basic qualities that help us to listen effectively: empathy, acceptance and genuineness. Let's look at each of these in a little more detail.

Empathy

Daniel: I just cannot begin to say what it felt like when I was told I was HIV-positive ... I just wanted to die there and then ... my whole world had come to an end. What would people think of me? What would my parents say, and the people at church? I simply wanted to disappear – it was a nightmare!

Pastoral counsellor: Daniel, from what you've just said I can hear the pain you went through when you were given the test result. It was as if your whole world had come to an end and what made it worse was the fear of what people would think, especially your parents and people at church. How's that pain now?

To 'listen' means that we try to understand life from another person's point of view. This does not mean that we always agree with them. But it does mean that we try to recognize that this is how *they* feel or think. We call this *empathy*. Empathy is not the same as sympathy. People on the whole do not want someone to feel sorry for them, but to hear and understand them. Empathy helps us to listen in such a way that we get into another person's shoes and experience what it feels like to be them for a while.

Acceptance

If we are really going to listen to someone then we have to learn how to empty ourselves of judgement. We need the quality of *acceptance*. We all look into other people's eyes to see if we are accepted. This is particularly true of those infected by HIV/AIDS. Stigma and discrimination have caused them to fear coming out into the open, in case they meet rejection and condemnation. When we listen to another person's story and their anxieties we need to show them that we are not judging them: even if we do not approve, we can still accept.

> **Daniel:** I suppose with time the pain has got a little less. I'm HIV-positive and I can do nothing about that. My great fear was that people were going to ask me how I got the virus. Everyone thinks you've been sleeping around being immoral, especially people at church.
>
> **Pastoral counsellor:** I hear the fear Daniel, but I'm wondering if the only person who really needs to know how you got the virus is you. What is important now is how you are going to live with it.

Genuineness

To listen with love is not a game or simply a matter of skills. We need to be *genuine*. We have to be ourselves and to be honest in our responses and concern, otherwise people can soon realize that we are simply play-acting.

> **Daniel:** That's easy for you to say, but I'm the one who's walking around wondering what people might think if they really knew that I was sick because I had sex with other men! What do you think of a Christian, a pastor of the church, who's gay?
>
> **Pastoral counsellor:** Daniel, I can hear that what I think of you is important to you. You want me to be honest. I think you are very frightened. You're not only trying to cope with the knowledge that you have HIV but you're scared of what people will think if they knew you are gay. At the moment you need love and support. That's what I want to give.

Jesus is a model of empathy, acceptance and genuineness. And in addition to these core qualities he also manifests two others which are crucial: *respect* and *challenge*. Why did Jesus love so much? Because he never lost sight of the dignity of each person he spoke to. Jesus showed tremendous respect for each individual that he met. He honoured the 'image of God' within them. As pastoral counsellors who are touching the lives of those living with HIV/AIDS, we must be sensitive to the sense of stigma and discrimination that each one feels and experiences. Our respect is vital, though it does not come easy. At times we will be invited to listen to someone whose story we do not like or who we are inwardly judging. We have to learn how to show the deepest respect – to view them through the eyes of God.

This does not mean that we should not challenge people. Jesus certainly did. However, challenge does *not* mean arguing or telling people off. Challenge really means helping others to see the inconsistencies in their way of thinking, the wrong information they may be holding and any values and beliefs that are life denying. Our challenge, like that of Jesus, comes from care and love, as we desire the best for the other person. At root, challenges remind people to take responsibility for their own growth and well-being.

> Respect includes not only seeing the person as she is now but seeing too what she is in the process of becoming. It is not respectful to label people as 'problems', even when they see themselves that way.
>
> Ann Long, *Listening*

These qualities are made visible to the person we are listening to by the way we listen and respond – such things as the way we look at them or nod our heads at the appropriate time, refrain from interrupting them and ask for clarification or summarize what we have heard. In all these ways we show them that we have heard them and respect the opinions and feelings they have expressed.

Those involved in pastoral counselling must remember that the person they seek to help has basic rights:

❋ The right to speak and be heard
❋ The right to their opinion
❋ The right to defend their views
❋ The right to their religious beliefs
❋ The right not to talk

When we listen to another person's story we are looking into a living document. Every book, every document, has a history and needs to be read with care and understanding in order to arrive at an appropriate interpretation. The respect we show to someone's story requires that we do not try to judge or provide an interpretation that is not their own. We must *listen* to them, not fit them into our own preconceived ideas.

Do pastoral counsellors have their own opinions?

It is very difficult to be free from our own opinions. All of us see life and listen to others by means of our own opinions and experiences. We are forever busy interpreting what we hear. That is why one of the most important ways in which we can learn to listen to others is to have first learnt how to listen to our own story. Self-awareness is essential for all who are involved in a ministry of listening. As we will see, our ability to listen is itself 'infected' by the talk that is going on inside our own heads, and the interpretation we give to the words and gestures we observe. This is especially true in our contact with people living with HIV/AIDS. Reflect for a moment on the following questions:

❋ What fears, prejudices and unquestioned assumptions do you carry around in your own mind?
❋ How well informed are you about the ways in which the HIV virus is contracted?
❋ Do you understand how the virus can develop?
❋ In what ways have you thought out the place of faith in relation to the HIV/AIDS pandemic?

* When you come into contact with vulnerable people such as children, commercial sex workers, homosexual men, or people who have been raped or abused, how comfortable are you with their pain and life experiences?

How can I best use myself in pastoral counselling?

Before we can begin to understand other people, we need to try and understand ourselves. The desire to help is of course a very important aspect of pastoral counselling, but this desire alone will not be sufficient to bring about a fruitful helping and healing relationship. As we try to relate to other people we do so with our own particular strengths and weaknesses. We do not help others because we imagine ourselves to be perfect or without problems or difficulties. Neither do we seek to help others because we imagine that we have all the answers!

Useful questions
* What might be painful or unpleasant for me in listening to people who are HIV-positive?
* What would be my greatest discomfort?
* What are my thoughts concerning death or suicide?
* Can I listen without interrupting others?
* What would I do if I were listening to someone with whom I disagreed or disliked?
* How do I cope with other people's strong emotions?
* Have I sufficient knowledge about HIV/AIDS?
* Do I have people who will support me in this work?

As people who want to cooperate in the healing ministry of Jesus, pastoral counsellors recognize that they are themselves 'wounded healers'. This awareness encourages them to be careful and sensitive so that they do not become 'wounding healers', infecting others with more confusion, anguish or self-doubt. It is never sufficient that we simply 'mean well'. We need to do the best we can through self-knowledge and to use ourselves wisely in the process of healing. Anyone who wants to enter a ministry of listening must first pause to consider how well they know themselves. What is it within their particular character that could help to facilitate or hinder a relationship of listening love?

The pastoral counsellor desires, above all, to create a relationship of trust so that the person being listened to feels free to talk. As a pastoral counsellor we are for a time trying to put ourselves into the shoes of the person who is at present sharing their story. This is far from easy because all of us filter what we see and hear through our own values, attitudes and beliefs.

This is why empathy, acceptance and genuineness are skills that we need to practise. To counsel is not therefore to sit in a position of superiority and then provide the answer; rather, it is to enter into a conversation, a dialogue, in which the pastoral counsellor seeks to understand what is being said so as to gain greater understanding and focus for the person.

To listen in this way is not as easy as we may think. It is an art and discipline and it requires us to be aware of our own personal prejudices, so that the living human being to whom we are listening may slowly unfold their mystery and find their truth.

As pastoral counsellors we encounter a person living with HIV/AIDS at a very vulnerable stage of their life. The issues raised and the feelings and thoughts that may well accompany them are very raw and call for great sensitivity. We are dealing with matters concerning life and death. We may even need to face and explore thoughts of suicide, anger, despair and the desire for revenge. Hence, we need to be aware that our first task is to assist the person to achieve greater emotional health and balance.

How can I help myself as a pastoral counsellor?

We need to be very practical and realistic. Being involved with pastoral care and counselling is extremely stressful. It is not easy to listen to people when they are in distress, nor see people each day who are suffering and for whom one cannot provide an immediate solution. Because the work is demanding, it is necessary to make sure that we too have someone with whom we can talk without breaking the trust of those whose stories we have received. For example, we can come together as a group of pastoral counsellors and share common problems and reflect on important issues. We can also find a trusted individual with whom we can clarify our ideas and attempt to build on our strengths and lessen our weaknesses.

Before we begin as pastoral counsellors it is as well to consider these few questions:

* Is there someone I respect and trust with whom I can share my experience of pastoral counselling from time to time?
* If I do talk with another person or group, how will I respect the confidentiality of those whom I am journeying with?
* How often do I think I might need to 'off load' – once a month, or simply when I feel stuck, overwhelmed, angry or confused?
* What are the qualities I look for in someone to listen to me? Do I possess these same qualities?

It is important to think about these questions, and the others we have already considered, *before* we volunteer for the work of pastoral counselling. After reflection we may realize that we are better suited to offering pastoral care rather than counselling. We need to explore what is required of us as a pastoral counsellor before plunging into something that will bring us a great deal of stress. The more we understand ourselves, the more we will be available to others and the more we will be able to manage the inevitable difficulties we encounter.

In the ministry of Jesus we see the importance of self-care. He often found time to be alone, as well as having time to be with others in their difficulties. Jesus tries at all times to listen to God (John 8:28). There is a rhythm of giving and receiving: he listens to people not only through their words but also in the very depth of their hearts (John 2:5; Luke 7:39, 40).

Read Mark 1:29–45

The fever left her and she began to wait on them ... Jesus healed many various diseases ... very early in the morning, before daylight, Jesus got up and went to pray

Jesus not only listened to others, but he also listened to himself!

How can listening to myself help others?

In a world where millions of people are in great need because of the HIV/AIDS pandemic, it might sound strange to be told that it is important to listen to oneself. Is this really a necessary preparation for listening to others? The simple answer is yes.

As we practise self-reflection so we can become increasingly aware of God's hand upon us throughout our life. The psalmist recalled with a sense of wonder that his actions, thoughts, moods, comings and goings, past and present were all known to God, whose hand had been upon him from his earliest beginnings in the womb (Psalm 139).

Ann Long, *Listening*

We are invited to 'search out your hearts and be silent' (Psalm 4:4). We are to 'examine our ways and test them' (Lamentations 3:40). So it is easy to understand why Jesus withdrew from time to time to a lonely place in order to reflect on his ministry and mission. This time of self-reflection and prayer enabled him to listen to the real needs of those who came for help.

In the end our personal growth is not just for ourselves, but for others and for God himself. If I want to listen fully and compassionately to other people and their stories then I must do the same for myself.

Henri Nouwen, *Reaching Out*

As we grow in understanding of ourselves at different levels of our thinking and feeling, we grow in understanding of others. If we stop and think for a second we know that we talk to ourselves nearly all day long. We carry inside us many voices, some of which we share with others, while others are kept secret inside. These voices express our likes and dislikes, our hopes and fears. As we learn to listen to our own story in the making we become more sensitive to the stories of other people, as well as to the presence of God in our life.

In summary, we can help ourselves to help others by:

* *Being informed* about HIV/AIDS and the issues involved for those affected.
* *Being non-judgemental.* Learn to listen to what is being said and not make a judgement about whether you like or approve. Whether we agree with what we hear is not the issue; it is someone else's opinion, not ours.
* *Being sensitive and compassionate.* This is just the opposite of feeling sorry for someone. We do not ask questions out of curiosity or to fill a silence. We ask questions in order to create a relationship of trust and to lead someone to greater understanding. Because we respect them we are willing and ready to stand with them in their difficulties.
* *Creating a loving environment.* If we are accepting of others they will feel able to open up. The safe environment we create will itself become a healing space.
* *Giving ourselves time to prepare before we meet with someone.* This will involve prayer and reflection to make a space within yourself so that you are free to receive what others would like to explore.

I had arranged to meet Jim at around 10 o'clock, but he was late. Suddenly, the door banged open. 'Sorry I'm late, you're probably angry and too busy to see me right now!' He said all this before I had a chance to say hello or even stand and hold out my hand. 'Shall I come another time?' His voice trailed off and his eyes were still looking at the ground.

'No, why do that? I've time now. Come in and sit down.' As I said this I walked towards him and took him by the hand. 'How's the family?' I said. "Those children of yours are really growing fast and are full of life.' He smiled and relaxed a little. 'Yes, they're all fine and even the business is picking up … I've nothing to complain about really.' Although he said this, his voice was flat and his face did not seem to match the good news he was sharing. He seemed anxious, as if there were a great deal on his mind.

There was a silence for a while. Jim seemed to be struggling to know where to begin. After some time I said: 'Jim, you say that there is nothing to complain about and that everything's fine, but you look as if there is a great weight around you. What's wrong?'

There was a big sigh and then he took me on a tour of his last few weeks. He explained that he had not been feeling too well recently and could not shake off a cough that seemed to have been around for months. He had got behind with work, and his energy levels had certainly dropped. That's why he had not been to church these past weeks: he simply had to catch up on the paper work while the house was free and the family were out. Then three weeks ago one of the men he worked with and travelled with on business had died. He had been ill for some time and had lost so much weight he seemed like skin and bones. That had really got to him. 'We were really good friends and had gone all over the world together on business trips, done all kinds of stupid things when we were away.' Because he had felt so unwell he could hardly sleep at night even though he was very tired, so he had taken himself off to the doctor's. 'The death of Richard had really frightened me … made me think, what if, what if I'd picked up the same thing. As I say, we'd done some pretty silly things when we were away.' Jim became silent again, but looked straight at me.

* If you were the pastoral counsellor how would you react now?
* What questions might you ask to help Jim share more of what is troubling him?
* What feelings and thoughts are going through your mind as a result of what Jim has said?

> Healing means, first of all, the creation of an empty space where those who suffer can tell their story to someone who can listen with real attention.
> Henri Nouwen, *Reaching Out*

A Way of Christian Listening

This chapter answers the following question:

✳ *Does Jesus give us an example of how to listen?*

Listening, like any worthwhile ministry, is tiring. It calls for concentration, commitment, faith, a putting aside of one's own preoccupations. As we listen in depth to another person we can be left feeling weary, depleted, sometimes anxious. How can we give ourselves generously yet remain resourced?

Ann Long, *Listening*

HIV/AIDS is an important challenge and invitation for all Christian communities to learn how to listen more effectively to those who are infected and affected. Listening to people living with this virus will help us to understand first hand what their real needs are, rather than assuming that we know ourselves what is best for them. Often, we think that listening properly will mean that we have to acquire certain skills and that these in themselves will help people to share freely the difficulties they are undergoing.

Maria, from inner-city Dublin, contracted HIV through intravenous drug usage. 'I used to think there was no point in coming off drugs because I was going to die anyway' was her comment on 23 years of drug and alcohol abuse. But now that she has been off drugs for 20 months, Maria, who looks younger than her 41 years, is anxious to press home the message that she believed drugs would kill her before HIV, for which she tested positive in 1985.

Maria has spent much of her life in and out of prison, as she depended on petty theft to buy her drugs. Her son (now 18) lives with her mother and her 12-year-old daughter is with foster parents. Maria says of her daughter: 'I can't give her the quality of life she deserves. But I want her to know that I love her unconditionally, enough to give her away. She may know that already – she's very loyal to me.'

Despite all the pain, Maria describes herself as a happy person who likes to make people laugh. She is tremendously supported by her Christian faith and by the staff of AIDS Care Education and Training in Ireland. 'I believe I have a future, whereas before I didn't. I'd like to be a journalist and write about how Dublin has changed. And I want women to know that they can still live with HIV.'

Christian Aid, *Women's Lives: Stories for World AIDS DAY 2004*

As Christians who desire to give time in order to listen, our real starting point is not so much skills and techniques (we'll talk about these in the next chapter), but rather a ministry – one that can be encouraged and practised in every community of faith, so that we can, as Christ's body, be fully open to the needs that surround us. To be aware of the needs of others requires sensitive ears and open hearts. We are, after all, trying to listen with genuine love and compassion and so our ministry of listening, like that of Jesus, is chiefly one of service.

Jesus, in the example he gives, shows that his prime motivation is to stand alongside others in their difficulties (Luke 7:11–17; 13:10–17; 17:11–19). He had come to 'serve and not to be served' (Mark 10:45). Hence, if we desire to serve as a pastoral counsellor, we will need to see it not simply as an activity requiring skills alone, but a way of supporting people so as to be a 'sacrament of love and compassion'. Listening may not seem a very practical or spectacular way of helping others, but it is a way of washing people's feet (John 13), following the example of Jesus: 'Love one another. In the same way that I have loved you ...' By making ourselves available for this ministry of listening we reveal deep compassion and great respect. We listen with and through love. It is this love that invites us to make ourselves available to stand alongside others in their need.

In her book *Listening* Ann Long says there are three images that are very important and which experience has taught her to be core elements in a ministry of listening love: gift, hospitality and healing. To be listened to, no matter how long or short a time, is indeed a *gift*. We are aware of this gift because we feel heard. This in turn gives us the important message that we have value. Jesus had the ability to make everyone to whom he listened or in whose presence he was to feel special. He acknowledged their dignity.

Likewise, to offer to sit down with someone while they tell their story is a visible way of showing *hospitality*. Like Abraham in Genesis 18:1–9, we welcome others and make them feel safe and at home. We create a sacred space. We receive another person as they are and not as we think they should be. Jesus offered to others a space where they could say what was troubling them. He did not offer the solution before the problem was voiced (Mark 10:46–52).

> Listening is the highest form of hospitality of the sort that does not set out to change people but to offer them space where change can take place ... hospitality is not a suitable invitation to adopt the lifestyle of the host, but the gift of a chance for the guest to find his own.
>
> — Henri Nouwen, *Reaching Out*

As we serve those living with HIV/AIDS we need first to create a space for them to talk freely about the difficulties that confront them. If we are indeed generous enough to offer hospitality to another person through our listening, though we will find it demanding, we will also find that we too receive a great deal.

If listening really is a gift and a way of showing hospitality, then it is undoubtedly a means towards healing. Each of us carries within ourselves a great deal that is often hidden away and undisclosed. When someone gently allows us to expose an inner wound, we generally feel relief. To see acceptance and genuine understanding in the eyes of another person is the beginning of a healing process. As Jesus made his way through Galilee and the surrounding districts he was simply 'present' to those who needed him most. It was this presence and service which were certainly a gift and a form of hospitality that brought about deep healing.

Yet listening is not something that is easy – it does not, as some might think, come naturally. Each day we hear many sounds and have the ability to distinguish words, but real listening goes much deeper than simply registering noises with our ears. As someone once said: 'I know you think you heard what I said, but what you think you heard is not what I actually said.' Much can go amiss between the one who is speaking and the one who is receiving!

Before we go into any more detail about listening as a key skill in pastoral counselling, let's turn to Jesus to see if he can give us any more clues about the way we can listen to others.

What example does Jesus give of how to listen?

If Jesus is our model in terms of compassion and care, then he is certainly a clear guide when it comes to listening with love. In order to discover a Christian way of listening, let's look at the story of the journey Jesus took with his disciples to Emmaus (Luke 24:13–45). The story is not only a marvellous example of our journey of faith – a journey from fear to joy, despair to hope – but it also provides us with a wonderful example of how Jesus accompanied others.

'While they were talking' (Luke 24:13–16)

The story itself gives no indication of how long the two disciples had been walking before Jesus joined them. They are deep in conversation as they walk together – so deep that they do not pay any attention to the stranger who has started to walk with them. The crucial point for us to remember here is that their journey began *before* the Lord joined them.

As Christians who desire to share in the ministry of Jesus by listening with love, we must always be sensitive to the fact that we are joining others on *their* particular journey. People have generally travelled quite a distance long before we come alongside them. Initially, we may not know how long they have journeyed. We may have no understanding of the joys and sorrows they have encountered on the way. Hence, it is of great importance how we begin to join them. We need to come alongside them with respect and humility.

As we begin to walk with others we need to be sensitive to what has gone on before. We adapt our rhythm to their pace and we tune into where they are. Jesus did not start talking straight away. He tried to see where the disciples were in their conversation and in their journey of faith. His task was not to divert them, but to affirm and acknowledge where they were in their understanding so as to help them gently to move on.

> If I can provide a certain type of relationship, the other person will discover for themselves the capacity to use that relationship for growth and change and personal development will occur.
>
> Carl Rogers, *On Becoming a Person*

There is always a temptation to fit people into a certain mould. We cannot assume that we know exactly what the person living with HIV/AIDS will be feeling or needing. We do not know what kind of experience they have had since learning of their status or that of a relative or friend. Jesus made sure that he got close to the disciples before he began to ask questions. If we begin by respecting others this will help us to become more observant and to learn from them so as to better understand.

Our first task as a pastoral counsellor is to develop a relationship. We may well feel tempted at first to ask ourselves: 'How can I help this person?' As we grow in listening with love, we will learn to ask a much more essential question: 'How can I provide a relationship that this person can use for their personal growth?'

Each conversation is a new start and a fresh opportunity to grow in understanding. To listen with love is to listen for the presence of God in a person's life and experience. We are standing on holy ground.

'What are you discussing?' (Luke 24:17–24)

The gospel story does not say why the disciples stopped speaking, but Jesus waited patiently until there was a pause in the conversation. He then asked them a simple question. In fact he had to ask them twice: 'What are you talking about?' This gave the disciples an opportunity to express the things that were really troubling them. In fact Jesus' question can be seen as having two important consequences. First, it allows the disciples to try to put into words their immediate experience. It is as if they relive what they have gone through. In other words the disciples are invited to *explore* their experience. This exploration provides them with an opportunity to voice what they were feeling and thinking as the experience was happening. It allows them to look at the interpretation they have given to a very significant event in their life.

Second, the very way in which Jesus asks the question focuses attention on the disciples. He does not fall into the trap of taking the attention to himself when they remark that he must be the only person in Jerusalem not to know what has been happening. He simply asks: 'What things?' He wants to hear from them the way they see things, rather than tell them straight away what really took place.

There is a saying: 'We had the experience but missed the meaning.' Talking with another person can be the occasion for us to recognize just what kind of meaning we give to the events we experience. A person living with HIV/AIDS may not have the chance to speak of their emotional, spiritual and psychological trauma. Jesus highlights another important quality of listening: he gave the disciples the one gift that would help them. He gave them his *presence*. When someone struggles to tell their story our first task is to be present to them, to give them our full attention. Hence, throughout our conversation, we try to keep our attention on the person and to focus the questions in such a way that it helps them tell their story fully. There can be no genuine understanding or change in outlook before their story is told completely.

For Jesus, the first stage in his listening with love is to *explore* the details of the story, to gather the information together. Perhaps for the first time the disciples are able to tell the story as a whole – what they had hoped for, but how they were disappointed.

'Was it not necessary?' (Luke 24:25–27)

It is very tempting when listening to others to interrupt and 'put them right' when we think that their interpretation of an experience is wrong. Jesus was more sensitive. He focused on the self-understanding of the two disciples. Then, through the careful use of scripture, he invites the disciples to explore and examine their feelings and thoughts. It is as if he opens up to them the possibility of an alternative interpretation. He encourages them to look at the experience recently undergone through the eyes of faith. Does this perspective give them a fresh understanding? He begins to strengthen their faith through scripture and slowly they begin to see their story through the story of God's presence and plan. Here we have the second stage in Jesus' example of listening with love. He leads others to a new understanding.

'He vanished from their sight' (Luke 24:28–35)

The final scene of our story provides us with several very interesting features. For a start, we do not know how long the three were in conversation. Local custom would have meant that as they were approaching the village and it was getting dark, then hospitality would have been extended to Jesus, but 'He made *as if* to go on'. Second, just as the eyes of the disciples were opened and they recognized him, 'He vanished from their sight'. Third, without regard for time or tiredness, the two disciples set out immediately to return to Jerusalem. There is in Jesus' accompaniment of the disciples a realization that he would not remain with them. He did not want to create a relationship of dependency. Rather, his great desire was to empower the disciples, to help them, as it were, to stand on their own two feet. His presence gave them the strength they needed. Hence, they could walk back to Jerusalem, to the very place from which they had wanted to escape.

In our role as a pastoral counsellor we can bring many different gifts, skills and techniques:

* We guide
* We encourage
* We support
* We provide compassion and presence

Above all, we are sensitive to the fact that as a companion on the journey of faith we cannot live another person's journey for them. We stay alongside them for an agreed amount of time and once our task is done we too can vanish until they should need us again. We help them to focus on the resources that they have within themselves and the Lord who gives them strength. In the story of Emmaus, Jesus has provided for us a simple model of listening:

Explore ➔ Understand ➔ Act

Because the disciples were given the time and opportunity to explore the story of their painful experience, they were led to a fresh understanding, which gave them the motivation for action. Jesus travelled with the disciples. In a ministry of pastoral counselling with those who are living with HIV/AIDS, we too are invited to accompany and travel with others on their journey towards wholeness. To journey with others is always then a sacred privilege and responsibility.

Although we have broken up the story of the disciples' journey to Emmaus in order to highlight Jesus' way of listening with love, in reality we cannot do this. The story in Luke's gospel allows us to appreciate that listening to others means a willingness to travel with them which requires:

* Respect.
* Recognizing the uniqueness of each person.
* Sensitivity to the fact that each person's journey began long before we came into their lives.
* The need to put aside our own assumptions about what this person needs.
* Learning how to be present and through our attention to facilitate the telling of their story.
* The story should be seen in the context of faith.
* The importance of the relationship that we create and the relationship we point to with God.

I was diagnosed as being HIV-positive more than nine years ago … I enjoyed excellent health, until the middle of 2002. I started to lose weight rapidly, and felt increasingly weak … The hospital possessed state of the art technology. I have no doubt that I owe the fact that I am alive today to this medical intervention. However, I did not flourish, and remained weak … After two weeks I asked to be transferred to a hospice run by nuns. They did not have the advanced medical equipment or the highly qualified staff. But they embraced me with love, and treated me with care and compassion. And my body immediately responded.

I know that I owe my own recovery entirely to the compassionate care and love that was given to me. We often think that the success of our work is measured by the amount of funding we raise, or by the amount of action we take … caring begins with 'attentiveness linked with love' and the best possible response may be to simply be there and stay with the person who is suffering.

Stuart Bate, *Responsibility in a Time of AIDS*

Listening with Loving Attention

This chapter answers the following questions:

* Do we really need to learn how to listen?
* What is there to learn about listening?
* What are the basic counselling skills that will help me to listen?
* What is active listening?

Globally, nearly half of all persons infected between the ages of 15 and 49 are women ... Because of gender inequality, women living with HIV/AIDS often experience greater stigma and discrimination ... AIDS is likely to be with us for a very long time, but how far it spreads and how much damage it does is entirely up to us.

Peter Piot, UNAIDS, *2004 Report on the Global AIDS Epidemic*

Listening, as we saw in chapter 4, was fundamental to the healing ministry of Jesus. It is no less important to our ministry in pastoral counselling. This chapter explores some of the basic counselling skills and techniques that will help us to be more effective in our ministry of listening.

Remember:

* This manual does not attempt to turn you into a professional counsellor; rather, its intention is to help you become more professional in the way you listen to others.
* The skills and techniques mentioned here are not meant to confuse you, but to give you confidence, so that you will feel more comfortable in your important pastoral ministry. See them as tools you can use in order to help others find inner peace and hope.
* At first they may seem strange, but with practice they will become part of how you listen. You will already possess many of these skills and be using them naturally. This chapter simply highlights them for you.

Most manuals concerned with counselling will use the phrase *active listening*. It's a phrase that may sound strange to us, as we seldom think of listening as an activity. That's why we hear people say things like: 'I didn't do anything, I just listened!' But 'just listening' is an activity. If we think about it carefully, when we listen properly we are in fact very busy people.

Do we really need to learn how to listen?

The simple answer is yes, because listening is not as easy as we may think. Just take a moment to reflect: in your experience how much hurt and confusion have been caused because people have misheard, misunderstood and misinterpreted what you have said? How much inner pain have you encountered because you have not heard correctly what others were trying to say? By and large, people do not listen. Instead, they 'fill in the gaps' or put words and thoughts into other people's minds and mouths.

To live with HIV/AIDS is already to live with the fear of being judged and rejected. Stigma and discrimination are real and they can often be more deadly than the virus itself. Yet the first stigma that people living with HIV/AIDS need to defeat is *self*-stigma:

* 'What are they saying about me?'
* 'What would they think if they were to know my status?'
* 'Are they washing that cup thoroughly because it's dirty or because I used it last?'
* 'Why do they avoid shaking my hand?'

We who desire to be a healing presence need to learn how to listen so that we do not cause more hurt by responding in a manner that is unhelpful. We need to learn how to listen so that we can best help someone tell their story openly and clearly. We need to learn how to listen so that we can begin to hear what is *not* being said among the many words that are spoken.

What is there to learn about listening?

Perhaps one of the first lessons about listening is that it involves far more than simply using our ears. Listening is more than hearing noises. It is one thing to hear the words that are spoken to us, and it is quite another to understand what those words mean. Hearing and listening are two very different things. When we hear, we are simply picking up sounds. When we listen, we try to make sense of what we hear. Therefore, when we listen to another person, we need to be aware of:

* Their tone of voice
* Their facial expressions
* Their body language

All these play an important part in communicating. So it's not simply what people say that is significant, but how they say it.

Our eyes as a partner in listening

Let's be honest, most of us listen through our mouths! That is to say, we already have a response playing in our heads before we've fully taken in what the other person is saying. Our eyes are very important aids to our ability to listen with understanding. Even before a person begins to speak, their body and their face are already communicating something to us.

As pastoral counsellors our own bodies can reveal what we are thinking and feeling about the person we are listening to, almost without us being aware. How we are present to another person is something we need to be aware of – without becoming too self-conscious about it! For example, looking at someone gives them the specific message that we are interested in what they are saying, but that does not mean we have to stare at them. We must be careful not to make others feel uncomfortable. Just as we look at others for signs of encouragement, so they too look at us. But what exactly are we looking for when we give our attention to someone?

Stop and think

Cast your mind back to a recent misunderstanding with someone else. Was it what they said that really upset you or was it the way they said it?

Feelings as a window into another person's world

As we look and listen we try to detect how the person is feeling. What emotions are their words trying to express? What emotions are being expressed by gestures and non-verbal communication? Notice the phrase 'trying to express'. Many people find it difficult to describe exactly how they're feeling, especially the first time of meeting. On the other hand, we will encounter others who have no problem in expressing themselves. So as we listen we try to note the feelings expressed and those that are somehow hidden beneath what is said and not said.

Music is a good example here. When we listen to music we often concentrate on the melody, but there are other things going on beneath it. In our pastoral counselling we try to pick out the different parts – tenor, base and alto – that go into the full story being told.

Stop and think

Can you remember an occasion when you were speaking to someone and they were busy looking over your shoulder or continuing to do what they were doing? How did that make you feel? What did you say to yourself about their behaviour?

Thinking as a trap

If we listen attentively, we will discover yet another layer of great significance *behind* expressed words and feelings. We will begin to hear what people actually think. When people say what is troubling them they also reveal what they think about themselves, others, the world at large and what they believe about God. These messages need to be heard in order to help us understand not only the issues that are being discussed, but also the context in which these difficulties live and move and have their being.

Stop and think

Reflect back on an occasion when you were trying to say something important to someone. How clear were you in what you said? Did you hope that the other person would pick up your real message without you having to spell it out?

Feelings   Thoughts   Tone of voice   Body language

Silence as a way of speaking

We express a great deal through words and body language, but we also need to listen to the times of silence, when a person stops talking. Is it because they have no more to say? Or are they stuck? Could it be that they've come to a point in the story that is very painful? Are they deciding whether to share some information or not? As pastoral counsellors we need to be comfortable with silence, while all the while trying to discern what the silence means. Silence, too, is a way of speaking.

Stop and think

Have you ever used silence as a way of communicating a message? How comfortable are you when people are silent and find it hard to say what is troubling them?

Our own inner noise

Finally, we need to be very conscious of how we ourselves react to what is being said. All of us filter what we hear through our own opinions, values and beliefs. We carry on a running commentary inside our own heads. We talk to ourselves, and this self-talk can prevent us from listening to others. If we fail to hear what the other person actually said and replace it with our own edited version, we are not helping the healing process at all.

Stop and think

If you are honest, how much do you listen to others and how much do you judge what you're hearing before you've heard the full story?

All these elements play a crucial part in our ability to listen. You see now why we are very busy people when we really listen and why it is called active listening. It is for this reason that people have turned to basic counselling skills to help them improve the quality of their listening.

What are the basic counselling skills that will help me to listen?

To be comfortable and effective Christian listeners we need to explore some of the basic skills that will help us as pastoral counsellors.

Active listening
This involves:
* Giving full attention to what is said and unsaid.
* Looking at the person when they speak.
* Reflecting back what they have expressed.
* Summarizing.
* Focusing the conversation.

Asking the right kinds of questions
We learn to ask open-ended questions that allow a conversation to flow.

Personal qualities
* Empathy
* Acceptance
* Genuineness
* Confronting
* Understanding one's own feelings and thoughts

Counselling model

Having some kind of structure or overall plan that helps the conversation move forward and come to some conclusion.

Problem solving

Helping people to devise some possible options and solutions.

Networking and supervision

Knowing where you can get help for others and obtain support for yourself.

None of these skills can or will replace the fundamental reason for entering upon a ministry of pastoral counselling. It is our faith that is of crucial importance. This belief in God prompts us to be people of compassion and to reach out to others. As we look at these skills, therefore, there is no need to feel nervous or to think that pastoral counselling has to be complicated. We will already possess many of the skills highlighted here, and be using some of them quite naturally. All we need do is look at these skills as ways of enabling us to do what we really want to do: to be channels of God's healing love.

So let's turn our attention once more to active listening.

What is active listening?

To listen actively means that we give another person our complete, undivided attention. As you can imagine, this requires a great deal of concentration. How can we do this?

1   By taking an interest in what the other person is saying.
2   By looking at the person and showing that we are following what is being said.
3   By using all our senses to pick up on verbal and non-verbal communication.

It is quite simple: the more we are able to show interest, the more another person will feel able to express themselves. When we listen actively we are a bit like a detective trying to pick up all the clues and information available. And if we listen carefully we will very often become aware that particular themes emerge time and time again. These themes reveal a basic pattern of thinking that can sometimes lie hidden behind the words.

Practical exercise

1   Take time to practise active listening with members of your family, friends and people with whom you work. Really show them that you're listening and give them your full attention. How easy do you find it? What reactions do you get?

2   Ask a friend to help. Find a time and space and then ask the friend to share an experience that was difficult for them to handle. Now reflect back to them what you think you heard them say, both in terms of the words and the emotions. Then reverse the roles. What was your experience like?

'I'm sure people at church are talking about me even though I've never told anyone I'm HIV-positive!' (Fear, suspicion, self-stigmatization)

'People are kind but no one seems to have any time to sit and listen.' (Loneliness, frustration)

'What kind of a mother lets herself be used in this way? I probably deserve being HIV-positive.' (Low self-esteem, blaming, anger)

'I know you'll think I'm evil, but I could really kill the person who gave me this virus.' (Anger, bitterness, resentment)

When Phyllis met Sister Florence at the clinic, she was desperate and ready to end her life after discovering that she was HIV-positive. 'Sister, I'm going to commit suicide … Life has become useless!'

Sr Florence looked up from the reception desk at the slim frail-looking girl before her. 'Well, before you do that, maybe you could just sit down and let me know your name and what's really troubling you … My name is Sr Florence and you …?'

'I'm Phyllis and you only have to look at me to see what's wrong. I have AIDS! So why go on living?'

'And so because you are HIV-positive and you feel very sick you want to end your life, is that it?'

'Yes of course that's it! I can't go on!'

Sr Florence then got Phyllis to tell the whole story from the beginning. As they talked, Phyllis began to see that life was not all bad. She also had to face the effect her suicide would have on her children and parents. She agreed to come to see Sr Florence each week at the same time. Meanwhile, Sr Florence gave her some medication to help.

When we listen we do so with an 'inner ear', listening not simply to the words of the story, but also to the underlying emotions that make up the total picture. We give our attention in order to enter, for a while, the world of another human being. We call this *empathic understanding* and it is the foundation and bedrock of active listening. We are listening so that we begin to understand more clearly the thoughts and feelings of the person. We want to know how they experience living with HIV/AIDS and the difficulties and challenges *they* encounter. Ultimately, however, it is not our understanding that is of crucial importance, but that our listening presence creates an environment which allows the person to understand their own feelings and thoughts.

There is a big trap that we need to be careful not to fall into. As pastoral counsellors we should take great care not to assume that we already know how another person is feeling or what they are thinking. Each of us is a mystery and must be treated with respect. As we listen we need to keep an open mind. The following skills will help us to do this.

* Write the word *assume*.
* Now draw a line on either side of the letter *u*.
* If we assume that we know what the other person is thinking or feeling, we make an ass out of *u* and *me*!

Questions to have in mind

A basic way in which we can help ourselves grow as listeners is to have in the back of our mind some simple questions to guide our listening and to help us understand more clearly the story we are being told.

Who? What? Why? When? How? Where?

These are questions that do not need to be asked outright as if we're interrogating someone! They form a mental checklist, although sometimes we may ask them in order to seek clarification:

* Why does this person need help at this particular time?
* What has happened that made them ask for help now?
* How long have they been living with this particular problem?
* What is it that they really want to express?
* Who or what has brought them comfort in the past?
* How have they coped with their problem up to now?
* Who forms their support network?
* What spiritual resources have they got or do they need?
* How best could I help them to help themselves?
* What is this person's problem?
* When and how did it begin?
* Who is involved?
* What are they looking for?
* How best can help and support be given?

These simple questions provide a kind of structure and framework for conversation.

Questions we speak out loud

Questions are never used simply to satisfy our curiosity, but to help the person who is telling their story to relate it freely and at their own pace. We ask a question so that:

* the story flows
* a point may be clarified
* the person themselves may gain a deeper understanding and meaning
* thoughts and feelings that lie hidden below the surface may be retrieved
* we convey that we are interested

Questions are a very important tool in our ministry of listening with love. Think of an iceberg. A great deal of an iceberg is hidden in deep waters and needs to be discovered with care. When someone begins to tell their story they only reveal a limited amount of information – the most important bits lie beneath the surface. The task of the pastoral counsellor is to help unearth these hidden bits so that a full picture is revealed. Our questions enable the person to explore, clarify and understand what they are really experiencing. We do not ask these questions simply to gather more and more information, but so that the person telling the story reaches a new level of understanding.

It is for this reason that we use what are commonly known as *open questions*. Open questions encourage people to reflect and respond in a deeper way to how they feel and what is happening. Open questions tend to have 'how', 'what', 'where' and 'when' attached to them. Closed questions require only a 'yes' or 'no' response and contain words such as 'was', 'is', 'did' and 'are'.

Practical exercise

Try making these 'closed' questions open:

﹡ When you were told that you were HIV-positive were you very upset?

﹡ Do you blame your husband now that you are HIV-positive?

﹡ Is your attitude to being positive acceptable?

﹡ Have you always had a problem of misusing alcohol and drugs?

﹡ Now you've been raped do you find it difficult to relate to men?

Clearly, we need to be sensitive about how we use questions so that people do not feel as if they are being interrogated or that we are prying into things that do not concern us. Pastoral counsellors have to be able to answer for themselves a crucial question: 'Why am I asking this question?' There is a real danger that when we feel nervous or stuck, or do not know what to say next, or there is a silence which we find embarrassing, we ask a question purely for the sake of saying something.

Questions are asked with a purpose in mind. We have to consider if *this* is the right time or place in our conversation to ask *this* question. What is the purpose of this question and what am I hoping to achieve? This important question is floating at the back of our minds as we listen.

Let's look now at some different types of questions and the purpose behind them.

There is an art and skill in asking questions that enables rather than diverts a person. To be on the receiving end of a string of questions can feel like being interrogated (e.g. 'So what did you tell your wife?' 'Then what did she say?' 'How did you react?'). It can be very distracting for a person to be continually interrupted by questions ... Ask questions sparingly and in order to help a person be more specific or to open up an area ... Often, as trust evolves in a listening relationship and the speaker is more forthcoming, the need for questioning will lessen.

Ann Long, *Listening*

Open questions rather than closed

Our chief desire as a pastoral counsellor is to provide time and opportunity for people to unburden themselves. We give them a chance to express what might have been locked away out of fear of being judged or misunderstood. When we ask a question in an open way, therefore, we give a person the choice as to how they wish to respond, whereas a closed question restricts their choice. We ask a question in a way that gives the person to whom we are listening the freedom to reflect and respond in their own way. Open questions *empower*.

> **Open-ended question:** 'Sarah, I wonder if you could tell me what your experience of going to the voluntary testing and counselling centre was like?'
> **Closed question:** 'Sarah, was your experience of going to the voluntary counselling and testing centre good or bad?'

Clarification questions

When people begin to share their stories they are often emotionally upset or confused. They are not always clear in the way they express themselves. We need to clarify what they mean by certain words or feelings. We cannot assume that we know what other people mean or how they interpret their own experience.

> **Clarification:** 'Sarah, when you say that going for testing and counselling was a nightmare, help me to understand what that means.'
> **Or:** 'Sarah, when you say that going for testing and counselling was a nightmare, it sounds like it was a pretty frightening experience. What was the most difficult thing?'
> **Elaboration:** 'Sarah, going for testing was far from easy. Could you say a little more about it to help me understand what it was really like?'

Specific detail questions

As we listen to others there will be times when we require them to be more specific about certain details of their story. We need sensitivity here because often people provide general descriptions in order to protect themselves.

How: 'Sarah, you said that it was the attitude of the person who gave you the results that made the experience difficult. How did their attitude come across?'

What: 'Sarah, when you said it was the attitude of the person who gave you the results that was so painful, what actually happened?'

Show me: 'You said that his attitude was so off-putting. Show me how he actually spoke and how that made you feel.'

When: 'Sarah, when did you first notice that his attitude was so difficult?'

Searching for meaning questions

Hidden behind everything we say is a whole system of values and beliefs that give meaning to how we see the world. As we listen to another person there are times when we need to check what personal meaning is attached to certain phrases and statements.

'Sarah, you said that finding out that you were HIV-positive made you feel unclean and punished by God. I wonder if you could say a little more about your faith and how you feel God looks at you now.'

'Sarah, what does this feeling of being unclean mean for you? Could you say a little more?'

'Punished by God? Could you tell me how your religious upbringing might have led you to feel like this?'

Searching for options and strengths

When people are in difficulties it is very easy for them to become focused on their problems to the exclusion of all else. Life seems heavy and without hope. One of the supports that a pastoral counsellor can offer is to help people recognize their strengths and hopes, and to encourage them to build on these, however small. Being HIV-positive or caring for a relative, family member or friend who is HIV-positive is one thing; the next step is to decide how to live with the virus. As with any other problem, we can focus on the difficulties or we can attempt to look for possible solutions and options. As we listen with love, we try to help people move forward from being weighed down with a problem to managing their difficulties resourcefully. We can empower people with questions that invite them to look for options and strengths.

'Sarah, you've said just how difficult it was when you found out you were HIV-positive and how it made you feel abandoned by God and unclean, but tell me a little about how you feel now. Do you still feel life is without hope?'

'It was clearly very painful when you first learnt about your positive status. I wonder was there anyone or anything that gave you support or hope, Sarah?'

'Sarah, now you know you are HIV-positive, what options are open to you, do you think?'

'Sarah, you've talked a great deal today and I think you've found that a help. Would talking with others who are HIV-positive be a possible option for you in terms of support and encouragement?'

The ways we use questions will either block people and close them in on themselves, or they will help to set them free. In our ministry of listening with love we need to understand the importance and value of questioning. That means we need to be sensitive to a person's anxieties and vulnerabilities. We need to use tact in the way we ask a question, when we ask and how we respond to the answer. Questions give direction to our conversation and we need to have a sense of where we would like to go. We need to pay attention to what is omitted in the answers given to questions. What is not said can very often be of greater importance than what is. We also need to be sensitive to the volume of our voice and to our facial expressions.

Often, people need to be reassured that we are really listening and following the flow of what they are saying. So how else can we convey to a person that we are present for them?

Encouragers

As pastoral counsellors we try to provide a space where people feel safe, comfortable and able to express themselves. We can do this very simply by encouraging the flow of the conversation:

* We use eye contact to give the message that we are paying attention.
* We use phrases such as: 'Uh-hmm'; 'Tell me more'; 'OK'; 'Right'; 'Then what?'
* We nod our head at the right time.
* Our facial gestures match what we are hearing.
* We can even lean a little towards the person.

These small gestures give the important message: 'I am with you, please continue, I want to hear more.' Of course, they have to be natural, otherwise people soon realize that we are not genuine.

> People are more than the sum of their verbal and non-verbal messages. Listening in its deepest sense means listening to clients themselves as influenced by the contexts in which they 'live and move and have their being'.
>
> Gerard Egan, *The Skilled Helper*

Reflecting back, clarifying and summarizing

Three practical ways of seeking understanding and of entering into the thoughts and feelings of another person are by reflecting back, clarifying and summarizing. These simple techniques indicate that we are following what someone is saying and want to stay with them as they continue with their story.

Reflecting back

This provides a very clear indication that you have heard what someone has said, that you are not judging what they think or feel, and are trying to understand. It also shows your willingness to enter into 'their world' and see things as they do. When we reflect back we do not use the exact words we have heard, as if we were a tape-recorder or a parrot! Rather, we pick out certain phrases and we 'play them back' so as to allow the person to hear what we have heard in terms of feelings and facts. We reflect back in order to check if we have heard correctly:

* 'From what I've just heard it seems …'
* 'Have I heard you correctly? Did you say … ?'
* 'Am I right in thinking … ?'
* 'From what you've just said it's as if I heard you say …'

These are simple phrases that we can easily use in order to introduce our reflection back. Look at the following example:

> As a pastoral counsellor you have been asked to go to the hospital where a patient's relative is asking to see you. The relative is distressed and meets you outside the ward.
>
> **Frank:** I'm so glad you came. My partner Tom is dying. His parents will not come to visit if I am here, as they do not want to admit that Tom is homosexual and they say I've killed him by giving him HIV/AIDS. I don't know how to help Tom. I feel so lost and alone. They just don't understand that we love each other. I don't want him to die. What can I do? I haven't killed him. I don't know why I asked you to come because you probably don't like gays either!
>
> **Pastoral counsellor:** Frank, I appreciate that what I think about people who are gay is important to you. But I'm hearing a far more important issue just now: the pain and sadness you feel at losing someone you love and the sense of rejection you feel from others, especially Tom's parents. You clearly want to do something for Tom and you don't know what! But if it helps, let me reassure you that I'm not judging you for being homosexual and I certainly don't think you've killed Tom, so let's begin by you helping me understand a little more about you and Tom and how he came to be in hospital.

Reflecting back the feelings and thoughts of the person we are listening to, in our own words and without adding any judgement or opinion, helps them to feel valued, as well as giving them a chance to redefine what they mean. Try for yourself in the following example:

You have been asked if you would call to see a member of the church who needs a listening ear. Mary is relieved to see you and begins to talk about her daughter, who has returned from university ill.

Mary: It's really good of you to come. To be honest I just didn't know where to turn and I don't know how much longer I can hold it in. There is so much going round in my mind I feel quite confused and I don't know where to begin ... Anyway, let me just start. It's Patience, my daughter. She's a good girl and has been at university, in fact only another year to go ... *(Mary breaks down and cries)*

I'm sorry, you must think I'm a fool. Why cry over a daughter's last year at university? I suppose that's just it really, I'm frightened she wont be able to finish, that it's all been a waste of time, not to say money. You see she had to come home about a month ago as she was quite ill. In fact, I now know that she's been ill for some time and hiding it from me. Of course, I knew deep down that something has not been right for a long time, but I suppose I didn't want to admit it ... It's no good, I've just got to say it ... she has this HIV disease and now she's gong to die and I feel so angry and ashamed. What am I going to do?

How would you respond to Mary by trying to reflect back the feelings and facts you've heard?

Clarifying

Using the skill of clarifying is a crucial way of making sure that we really do understand what another person has said and how they are actually feeling. Clarifying means asking the person to explain a little further. A great deal of misunderstanding can be avoided by simply asking the person to say a little more about a particular point or to let you know if you have understood correctly. For example:

'Could you help me understand a little more, when you said ... ? What did you actually mean?'

'You said that you felt ... What exactly caused you to feel this way?'

'Could I just check something to see if I've heard you correctly? Did you say ... ?'

'I'm just wondering, when you first heard that your son has HIV, how did that make you feel?'

'Who did you want to tell first that you were HIV?'

'When you decided to tell your partner of your status how did he react and how did that make you feel?'

Once again, this simple technique gives a person the clear message that we truly want to understand fully what they are revealing. When we seek to clarify, we are saying in effect: 'I'm with you, help me to understand more.' When a person tells their story and reveals their feelings they are as it were opening a window into their world. Clarification seeks to acknowledge that people exist within different contexts, and that in order to understand them and their difficulties we need to be clear about the contexts to which they belong. The flow diagram gives some of the contexts that surround people living with HIV/AIDS.

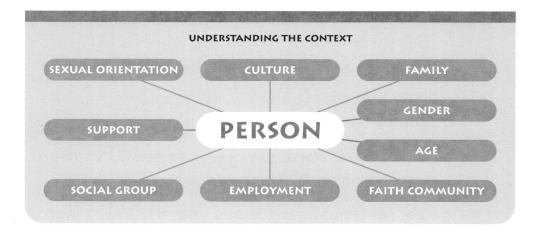

UNDERSTANDING THE CONTEXT

SEXUAL ORIENTATION   CULTURE   FAMILY

GENDER

SUPPORT   **PERSON**

AGE

SOCIAL GROUP   EMPLOYMENT   FAITH COMMUNITY

Let's go back to Frank and the pastoral counsellor at the hospital:

Frank: Tom and I have been together for nearly eight years. We met at a party and we seemed to get on from the beginning. I just can't imagine life without him ... he's all I've got. It was about a year ago that he began to feel ill and nothing seemed to make him feel better. Eventually, I persuaded him to go to the doctor and ask to be tested for HIV. We were devastated when the news came that he was positive. I nursed him at home until last week, when he simply had to come into hospital. All the nurses are kind, but I can see them looking. Why can't people see us as normal? That's what makes it so hard now.

Pastoral counsellor: Hard because if one of you were female then your relationship would be acknowledged and your present pain understood?

Frank: Yes, that's just it. If I'd come home with a girl on my arm and she was now seriously ill my family would be supportive. But now they're just ashamed. HIV/AIDS, well it's just what we deserve isn't it?

Pastoral counsellor: Frank, no one deserves HIV/AIDS, and it certainly isn't a judgement from God, so help me to understand a little more about why you asked Tom to go for an HIV test, what made you suspect?

Much of the misunderstanding and frustration that we experience in life can be due to the simple fact that although people hear our words they interpret them differently to what we intended. Clarification is crucial to prevent misinterpretation. In pastoral counselling it is necessary to understand people's stories as *they* understand them and experience them, not as we think it is.

Let's continue with the story of Mary and her daughter. What would you want to clarify in the following example? How would you phrase the questions?

> **Mary:** As I said earlier, I knew something was wrong for a long time. She just wasn't herself and didn't phone as much. Even when she did it was hard work trying to get any conversation from her. Not like when she first went to university – she loved it and was full of news, but something seemed to have happened to change all that. Well, now I know what it was … no wonder she was withdrawn. I'm so angry. Why didn't I do something when I saw she was unhappy … perhaps she wouldn't be so ill now, maybe she wouldn't be HIV-positive? Why couldn't she tell me something had happened? All these questions, they go round and round in my head.

Summarizing

When people begin to tell their story they often speak for a long time. The skills of reflecting back and clarifying can help break up this monologue into manageable sections. It can also be helpful at times to stop the person and try to pull together what you have heard. This is especially helpful towards the end of a conversation. A summary tries to state simply and clearly what has been expressed in terms of feelings, facts and themes, and the bare outline of the problems and issues raised. One of the most useful things about summarizing is that it helps move on the conversation – this is especially true if a person is not very clear in the way they express themselves, or if they go round in circles, simply repeating the story again and again. Summarizing can help break this kind of rambling and provide an opportunity for greater understanding. There are at least four basic ways we can try to summarize:

1   As simply as possible we can describe what has taken place in the conversation so far in terms of details and feelings.

2   We can ask the person to make a contrast. Summarize what has been said, then ask the person to contrast either:

*   *the past with the present:* 'You were saying that when you first were diagnosed with HIV you felt that your life was over. I wonder if anything has changed … how do you feel now, at this moment?'

*   *the present with the possible future:* 'You say that at present you feel you can't face going back to work in case people find out that you are HIV-positive. Tell me a little about what the advantages might be of being back at work.'

*   *the past with the future:* 'You were very angry with God and ashamed when you first learnt that your son was HIV-positive and you said you wanted to hide. Tell me how you would want to relate to God and your son in the future now that you've grown in understanding.'

3   We can ask the person to choose what is most important. Often, when people talk, particularly in the beginning, they lump a lot of issues together, and everything comes out at once. We need to check which issues they want to discuss, rather than what we assume to be important. For example:
'You've said quite a lot and I'm wondering from the things you've just told me – *a, b, c, d, etc.* – which of them you'd like to explore first.'

4   By means of our summary we can tentatively suggest an issue that seems to be uppermost in the person's concerns:

'From all that you have just told me – a, b, c, d, etc. – I'm left wondering if issue b is the one causing you most discomfort at present. Is this the one you would like to talk more about?'

At what point in our conversation we decide to summarize is up to us to discern sensitively. Some pastoral counsellors like to summarize:

* At the end of the conversation.
* At the start of the next conversation.
* When giving someone something to reflect on before the next encounter.
* In order to identify the major problem/issue.
* When there is confusion.

In tuning in to a person we will sense when it is necessary to pause and summarize.

Focusing

The final active listening skill to highlight here is focusing. We have already mentioned that people are often not very clear or focused when they begin to talk. This is particularly true at the beginning of the very first meeting. It can make life difficult if you are trying to listen:

* What is this person really saying?
* What's really bothering them?
* What should I pick up on?

These are important questions to have at the back of our mind as we listen with genuine love and compassion. Look at this example from Mary, whose story we have met before:

> **Mary:** I know it was unchristian of me, but I lost control when my daughter first told me she was HIV. I've always had a problem with my temper. I was so angry with her, with God, with myself. I felt let down. Why couldn't she have told me earlier? Right now I feel so ashamed of myself and I don't know how to approach her.

What do you pick up on? How would you respond? There are many general remarks that need clarification and exploration. In order to do this you need to know where you want Mary to focus. Do you:

* *Focus on the feelings?* I was so angry. I felt let down. I feel so ashamed.
* *Focus on the thinking that lies behind the feelings?* It is unchristian to lose my temper. My daughter should have told me earlier. God should not have let this happen. Why has he done this to me/my daughter? I have failed as a mother. How can I face people? HIV is a punishment.
* *Focus on the problems?* The Christian response to anger. Anger management. Her understanding of HIV. Her image of God. Her relationship with her daughter.
* *Focus on possible solutions?* How she could approach her daughter. Where is she going to find spiritual and practical support? Ways of dealing with anger.

To focus needs real discernment and practice. We need above all to be sensitive. We should not fall into the trap of focusing on what appeals to us, but on what would best help the person find freedom and inner peace. We focus in order to bring greater clarity. People sometimes make general remarks: 'It was unchristian of me', 'I feel so ashamed of myself.' In focusing we try to turn these general remarks into more specific ones, so that the person grows in understanding and finds a way through. Here is one way that a pastoral counsellor can try to move Mary forward by combining the skills of summarizing and focusing:

> **Pastoral counsellor:** Mary, could we just pause there? You have expressed a lot in what you have just said – about feeling let down by God and your daughter, feeling angry with yourself and God, having problems with anger and now being stuck in knowing just how best to approach your daughter. I don't want to lose anything of what you've said, but could we just focus for a little on what it was about her telling you about being HIV that made you so angry?

Perhaps you could think of another approach.

In this chapter we have looked at a few of the basic counselling skills that will help us to listen more effectively. With practice and reading you will discover more such skills. For now, we will turn our attention to the help that having a structure might have for our listening with love.

A Process that Helps Us to Heal

This chapter answers the following questions:

✳ *Why does our pastoral counselling need a structure?*
✳ *Can you suggest a structure?*
✳ *How can this structure be summarized?*
✳ *What about confidentiality, support and networking?*

All who embark upon and continue the practice of pastoral counselling will make mistakes, as well as enjoy successes. Training for counselling is an ongoing process. Books can only take us so far. Each new person seen adds to the experience and learning … Through the careful use of his/her own thoughts and feelings, through listening to the 'still small voice' within themselves and in the other, the pastoral counsellor will find that this particular way of being alongside people in need brings emotional, intellectual and spiritual fulfilment.

Michael Jacobs, *Still Small Voice*

Counselling, as we have already mentioned, can simply be defined as a conversation with a purpose. If this is true, then our conversation as pastoral counsellors with those living with HIV/AIDS will benefit from having a simple structure. Of course, this does not mean that it has to be formal or inflexible. Instead, it means having a clear aim and goal. Our aim is to make ourselves available so that those needing to express themselves can do so freely and openly. The goal of our conversation is that the person can explore what is troubling them and move towards being less burdened and more equipped with confidence and ways of coping. We hope that the other person will come to feel able to face their difficulties with renewed strength. With this in mind let's look at a simple counselling structure that might help us achieve our purpose: to help others help themselves.

Why does our pastoral counselling need a structure?

As pastoral counsellors we have a genuine desire to be of service. We want to participate in the healing ministry of Jesus through our active listening to those living with HIV/AIDS. Having a clear and simple framework in the way we listen increases the therapeutic value of our ministry. The story of Jesus' journey with the disciples from Jerusalem to Emmaus (chapter 4) revealed the structured way in which he led the disciples to a new understanding and interpretation of their experience.

While it is true that 'a problem shared is a problem halved' we can help with greater effectiveness if we have some kind of inward plan that gives shape to our conversation. This is not the same as saying that we already have a solution or a fixed process that everyone has to go through. Rather, we are suggesting that a structure gives shape to the way we listen and allows for greater flexibility. Having some model or framework in mind protects and helps people to feel confident, as they sense some kind of movement from A to B. It also protects the pastoral counsellor: it reminds us that we are not there to solve other people's difficulties, but to help and encourage them to find ways of solving their own problems and to discover their own inner resources.

At the age of 41 Pearl was diagnosed HIV-positive at a government hospital in Durban. She received no counselling before or after her test. 'I felt as though I'd just been given a death sentence. Fortunately, I was with my mother and sister, but they were probably more shocked than I was. We went home and had a few drinks and I threw some things around the house.'

Pearl's health deteriorated: she developed thrush, ear infections and night sweats. Worse still, neighbours in the block of flats where she lived put up posters on the wall outside: 'Don't touch Pearl, she's got AIDS.' Her teenage children suffered enormously.

'My son used to take the posters down on the way to school, but it affected him a lot. He took drugs and neglected his school work. My daughter rejected me completely.'

Pearl's mother picked up a leaflet about Hillcrest AIDS Centre and rang for assistance. A nurse called with one of the voluntary counsellors. 'You expect a Christian organization to treat you like a human being, and they certainly did do that. Cheryl and I never pray together, but I do pray for her. And I believe in miracles. I mean, the fact that I've lived to become a grandmother is a miracle, when I think how sick I was a few years ago.'

G. Williams and A. Williams, *Journeys of Faith*

People need to express themselves for a variety of reasons. Some simply want to pour out their troubles and then go away relieved, while others are stuck and do not know how to move forward. Having some framework in mind enables the pastoral counsellor to help a person gain perspective and frees them from getting lost in their own stories. Structuring our listening also prevents the pastoral counsellor getting lost!

There are many counselling models, each emphasizing a particular approach. This manual suggests a possible framework that picks the basic ingredients from a great variety of helpful models. With practice and further reading you will find and refine your own method of listening with love.

> Clients come to counselling in pain, with problems, with decisions, in crisis and in need of support. They need to relate to or become connected to counsellors as a way of working on their concerns. I define the counselling relationship as the quality and strength of the human connection that counsellors and clients have ... Listening and showing understanding ... are central to building quality relationships with clients.
>
> Richard Nelson-Jones, *Practical Counselling and Helping Skills*

Let's list these basic ingredients now and then take a brief look at each in turn:

1   Prayer and preparation
2   Building a relationship of trust
3   Exploring the present situation
4   Understanding what is going on and how to move forward
5   Planning for action and setting goals
6   Reviewing strengths and building on them

Prayer and preparation

We may never have thought that listening needed preparation, but then we may never have thought that there was so much involved in listening!

We see in the example of Jesus that he often went to a lonely place in order to pray, especially before important events. He needed time apart to help him focus his attention. As people who want to listen with deep compassion, pastoral counsellors need time to pray, read and reflect. We need time to create an inner space so that we can be truly available and present to those who seek a listening heart.

Part of our preparation (alongside prayer) is to take time to inform ourselves about the variety of complex issues that surround HIV and AIDS. As pastoral counsellors we can often best be of service to others by giving them the correct information. To do this we must see to it that we are informed ourselves.

We need to be aware of the issues that may very well come before us as we make ourselves present to others through listening:

* Anger
* Fear
* Self-harm
* Rape
* Stigma
* Gender inequality
* Child abuse
* Shame
* Sexual orientation
* Blame

* Crisis of faith
* Difficulty with prayer
* Hatred and revenge
* Drug dependency
* Poverty
* Prostitution
* Blaming
* Forgiveness
* Domestic violence

These are just some of the difficulties that arise as a result of living with HIV/AIDS. We need to reflect on them and discover our own thoughts and feelings about them, so as to empower others. Not that other people need our thoughts, no, but if we have taken the journey we may be able to guide others along the way to finding their own answers.

If people have asked to see a pastoral counsellor then we bring to them in our listening service a belief in the presence and love of God. So let us begin with prayer – a prayer that already begins to create an atmosphere of acceptance and trust. Let us not be frightened of praying and inviting the person to pray. Much will be revealed as they express their hopes and fears. Prayer reminds us that we stand on holy ground and that there is a power greater than ourselves.

Building a relationship of trust

When we feel at ease with another person we often experience release from tension. The way we greet people, the volume of our voice and our facial gestures, convey a genuine warmth and acceptance. Of course, the reverse can equally be true! People, after all, are reading us even before we speak.

> Helping, at its best, is a deeply human venture. Models, methods, techniques and skills are tools at the service of this venture ... the relationship between helper and client is extremely important, but in the end it is a relationship of service, not an end in itself.
>
> Gerard Egan, *The Skilled Helper*

It is true that *how* we say things has a greater impact than *what* we say. Therefore, to use people's names in a respectful manner, to be sensitive to people's age, gender and culture, can be a clear way of affirming their identity and showing our respect for them.

When we first meet people we need to introduce ourselves: explain who we are and tell them our name. Even though they may have been the ones who asked to see us, we need to spend time breaking the ice. This can very often be done through simple 'small talk', which gives the message that the person is of value. The introductory moments of our conversation are a significant way of settling ourselves into this new relationship and allowing the person (as well as ourselves) to relax. This is especially important at our first meeting, but it is valuable in each encounter. The first moments we meet another person give us the opportunity to 'take the temperature' of our encounter.

American Episcopalian priest Margaret Guenther has written beautifully in her book *Holy Listening* about listening as a way of creating a 'sacred space'. Each time we encounter one another we need to be sensitive to entering that sacred relationship of encounter, not only with the human being before us, but also with the presence of God within each of us. We are touching the divine, so we need to learn how to acknowledge that by not rushing the initial moments when we try to 'connect' with the person who is in difficulties. Initially, we may feel that 'just chatting' is a waste of time, but we 'waste time' like this at the beginning so as to build a relationship of trust.

In a country in Asia a priest who was HIV-positive was withdrawn from his parish and from all diocesan activity and sent to a retreat centre hundreds of miles away, with no further contact from his diocese.

In the debriefing following a workshop exercise in Asia, several priests said that they could not tell their bishop if they discovered they had HIV. Humbly, movingly and with great affection, the bishop, also a participant, stood up and told the priests that if any of them was ever to find they had HIV, he would be there for them.

In a country in Southern Africa a person described a not-untypical scenario where the husband beat and raped his wife when he returned from the bar. When she finally appealed to the local priest to intervene she was told to go home and bear her suffering.

In a country of East Africa the local priest refused to visit a woman who had AIDS, because she had been a sex worker. When he heard about this the bishop himself visited the woman regularly until her death and celebrated her funeral Mass – a solemn requiem Mass – in the cathedral.

Ann Smith and Enda McDonagh, *The Reality of HIV/AIDS*

Strange as it might seem, even though someone has asked to see a pastoral counsellor, and they may desperately want to talk, once the time has come they often find it difficult to know where to begin. We can gently reassure them that this is normal and invite them to take their time and begin their story wherever it seems right to begin. Or we can prompt them by suggesting: 'Why not start by saying what made you decide you wanted/needed to talk with someone?' Conversely, we may meet people who will simply start talking as if the radio has been switched on or the dam wall has burst!

And now here is my secret, a very simple secret: It is with the heart that one can see rightly; what is essential is invisible to the eye ... It is the time you have wasted on your rose that makes your rose so important.

Antoine de Saint-Exupéry, *The Little Prince*

The thing to remember as we enter the world of another person is that the quality of our presence is of greater value and support than what we might say.

Exploring the present situation

If we recall the story of the journey to Emmaus we will remember that as Jesus joined the disciples he asked them to share their personal experience. 'What are you talking about?' he asked. 'The things that have happened in Jerusalem these past days', they answered. 'What things?' he replied. By means of this brief exchange Jesus was simply saying: 'Tell me what's bothering you … what's the problem?'

We can do the same at the beginning of our time of listening. We have come in order to give the person living with HIV/AIDS the time and opportunity to express their deepest concerns. We let them tell the story of this virus as they experience it. By our use of questions, reflecting back, listening presence, etc., we gain an initial understanding of what the issues are that they are struggling with. In our sensitive exploring we help clarify for them the most important concerns and begin to look for ways of coping.

Exploration skills
* Active listening
* Guiding questions
* Reflecting back feelings and facts
* Summarizing
* Clarifying
* Paraphrasing
* Focusing

Often, when people begin to talk, they present one issue, or a number of complex issues, as the problem, while the real problem is hiding beneath the surface. It is only as people talk and as they listen to themselves and are guided by a sensitive listener that they really begin to see what is truly troubling them. That is why our most helpful contribution is to allow the story to flow and then reflect back the feelings and facts we have heard. If the person doesn't seem to express any feelings while they talk we can perhaps gently point this out:

'You've told me how you broke the news to your parents that you were HIV, but I'm wondering how you felt about doing that, as you actually never mentioned it.'

Then, as we sense that the story has been told in full, at least in this first edition, we can ask something like this:

'Ruth, what is at the heart of all that you have been saying, what's most important?'

Our first task as listeners is to help people tell the story as it is.

Understanding what is going on and how to move forward

When we speak of understanding as a stage in the process of listening with love it is not so much that we as listeners grow in understanding (though this is important), but that the person who is sharing their story grows in self-understanding. Of course, we cannot give people self-understanding, but we can give them the time and opportunity that might allow it to come about. One of the most unhelpful things we can do as a pastoral counsellor is to say something like:

'I know exactly how you feel and I think this is what you should do!'

Or:

'Now it seems to me that this is your problem and I advise that you …'

These are just the kinds of responses that people do *not* need to hear and that block them from expressing themselves freely. It is often only through talking that people come to a deeper understanding of what is truly causing them pain. As we explore, the person says in effect: '*This* is how I see and experience being HIV-positive.' In active listening we try to act as a mirror and through reflecting back and clarifying we respond: 'I hear what you are saying, but is this the only way to see things? Is the interpretation that you are giving the only option?'

Skills of understanding
* Advanced empathy
* Confronting/challenging
* Alternative interpretations
* Use of self

Think back to an occasion when you yourself had a problem that really worried you. Could you honestly see things clearly? Maybe not. As a pastoral counsellor we're not simply sponges that soak up everything without challenging. Sometimes, as an outsider, we can see more clearly where people's thinking is leading to unhappiness. But our task is not to tell people they are wrong and how they should think. Our service of love is to try to help them discover for themselves where they are stuck. How can we do this? Let's look at some of the skills of understanding.

Advanced empathy

When we try to show empathy we try to enter the world of the person to whom we are listening. We allow ourselves to see things from their perspective. We reflect back to them the feelings and facts that we hear. But as we listen to others we become aware of unspoken feelings and thoughts that are only implied and hinted at. The person may well be aware they are hiding certain things or they may be unaware of it. As trust develops between us we can tentatively share these insights:

'It's almost as if you were saying …'
'You've never said that you are angry, but it's as if I can see it just below the surface.'
'As you describe your feelings the picture that comes into my mind is …'

Advanced empathy invites us to reflect back – at a deeper level – not our interpretation of what the person is saying but what is being half said or said in a confused way. So, as we listen, we ask ourselves:

* What is this person only half saying?
* What are they hinting at?
* What is being said in a confused way?
* What am I hearing behind the spoken words?

Let's go back to the story of Mary and her daughter who came home ill from university.

> **Pastoral counsellor:** Mary, you have said a lot about feeling angry with your daughter Patience and with God. You felt let down, ashamed. But unless I'm mistaken I can also hear underneath all that a sense of blaming yourself. It's almost as if I'm hearing you say: 'Where did I go wrong that my daughter couldn't come and speak to me sooner? Why didn't I do something when I saw her depressed? What kind of mother am I?'

As a pastoral counsellor we are partners in a process of understanding. We do not put words or ideas into people's mouths or heads. Rather, we check our hunches and intuitions. Acting as a mirror, we help the person to say more clearly what was expressed in a confused way, to bring out what is only half said and to look at what was revealed as a superficial thing in a deeper way. Empathy asks us to see the world from the perspective of the other person. Advanced empathy invites us to share a world beyond what is being said.

Confronting/challenging

We all suffer from selective vision and hearing. Not that we do this intentionally (at least, not all the time!). All of us have blind spots where our understanding of a situation and problem is not all that clear. In this stage of the helping process we try as a compassionate listener to help people arrive at new perspectives. This means that at times we need to challenge or confront them with the inconsistencies or unhelpful attitudes, values or patterns of behaving that we are sensing.

When listening to people who live with HIV/AIDS we are in the presence of people who are vulnerable. Already, they feel the effects of stigma and discrimination. They may well have external and internal negative voices which reinforce their sense of being a 'victim'. We therefore need to be sensitive as to how we challenge them. We are not there to tell people they are wrong. Instead, we are there to help them discover deeper understanding by recognizing for themselves the ways they think and act that are self-defeating.

Experience will teach us the areas that need to be challenged and confronted. Here are some things we need to challenge:

* A desire to blame others for their problems.
* A failure to take opportunities which might bring relief.
* A failure to be very clear about what is their real problem.
* A tendency to make excuses why they cannot change the way they think or feel.
* An interpretation of events that is not altogether true.
* An attitude that looks to others to solve the problem.
* Beliefs, values and attitudes that maintain unhealthy behaviour and problem situations.
* Talking about everything except the real issue.
* An unwillingness to think of possible solutions.

There are many others. We need to be on the look out as we listen. 'Where is this person not helping themselves to find inner peace and healing?'

Read John 5:1–9

Jesus simply asked the man: 'Do you want to be healed?' The question required a simple 'yes' or 'no'. The man on the mat could not see this and so began with his excuse: 'I have no one to put me in the water ...'

We are partners in the healing process when we are able to help others hear their own false and negative ways of thinking and acting. The truth sets them free to understand more deeply.

> **Pastoral counsellor:** Mary, you said earlier that you were angry when you found out from Patience that she had been raped by one of the lecturers and that is how she probably contracted the HIV virus. You spoke a lot about feeling ashamed and let down, disappointed in yourself and your daughter, not to say with God as well. I'm just wondering, though, what you could do to protect other girls from suffering the same violation and abuse?

Alternative interpretations

Victor Frankl was an eminent psychiatrist and professor at the Vienna Medical School who died in 1997. He was a survivor of Auschwitz concentration camp in the Second World War. During his imprisonment he witnessed many forms of hideous suffering, but never lost hope. In his book *Man's Search for Meaning* he makes the observation: 'Everything can be taken from a man but one thing: the last of the human freedoms – to choose one's attitude in any given circumstances, to choose one's own way.' The events of our life, whether they are experienced in the present or are memories of the past, do not actually impose their feelings upon us; rather, how we feel about a particular situation is largely determined by the way we 'choose' to interpret the events. We feel as we think!

> The prisoner who had lost faith in the future – his future – was doomed. With the loss of belief in the future, he also lost his spiritual hold; he let himself decline and became subject to mental and physical decay. Nietzsche's words: 'He who has a *why* to live for can bear with almost any *how*.'
>
> Victor Frankl, *Man's Search for Meaning*

When we try to help people imagine an alternative interpretation of the events they are suffering we are not playing a game of 'let's pretend'! As we listen to others, and indeed to ourselves, we become aware that the way that situations are described is not always the *only* way they can be understood. Sometimes we need to encourage people to look at possible alternative interpretations. For example, Mary in the story we have been using said as she began:

'It's no good, I've just got to say it … she has this HIV disease and now she's going to die and I feel so angry and ashamed. What am I going to do?'

As a pastoral counsellor journeying with those living with HIV/AIDS we need to give people proper information and challenge their misinterpretations. 'Is it true that because someone is HIV-positive they are going to die?' No, it is not. That we are all going to die eventually is of course true, but no one has to die because they have HIV/AIDS.

> **Pastoral counsellor:** Mary, I'd like to go back a bit in our conversation. When you first told me that Patience was HIV-positive you seemed to suggest there was no hope. If I remember correctly you said something like: 'She has the HIV disease and now she's going to die.' From what we've said about the virus and the needs of those infected, how true is that?

As we use this skill we try to invite the person to step back and look at what they have said and how they feel from an alternative perspective. In doing this we can bring into focus the person's own understanding of the Christian faith. How does the Christian story inform and influence their personal story? Jesus took the disciples with whom he was travelling on the Emmaus road on an inner journey – a journey through scripture – and their eyes were opened. In applying the healing ointment of the scriptures we can often find greater self-understanding and freedom.

Advanced empathy, challenging and looking for an alternative perspective are three very basic skills that can be used at this stage of the counselling process. There are others, of course, but these help the pastoral counsellor to help a person examine their reactions and responses to the events causing distress. They seek to look at a broader picture, so that a deeper understanding emerges.

Planning for action and setting goals

Action skills
* Problem solving
* Goal setting
* Role play
* Homework/reflection
* Evaluations and endings

At the heart of our ministry of listening with love is the desire to help others to live in a way that is more life giving. It is often true that simply having the chance to unburden themselves of the difficulties of life is enough for most people to feel some kind of relief and a new energy for life. As a pastoral counsellor, however, we also have the task of helping people to be practical and to work for new ways of living. We cannot solve people's problems; HIV/AIDS cannot be wished away. But perhaps the real healing is to look at the difficulties we face and to find ways to live with them. The Buddhists have a saying: 'The best way to rid yourself of an enemy is to make that enemy your friend!' The action stage of the healing process is not about taking problems away, but helping people to identify strengths so they can learn how to cope and adapt to life with HIV/AIDS.

Disclosing our status is one thing, but the person living with HIV/AIDS will need to be guided by the pastoral counsellor to identify coping strategies that will turn this life-threatening virus into a life-affirming choice. Once the person has told their story the goal is to give them the opportunity to ask and begin to answer the crucial question: 'Where do I go from here?'

The two disciples who walked with Jesus from Jerusalem to Emmaus were certainly not the same people by the time they arrived in Emmaus. Their eyes had been opened. When they returned to their friends they were very different. Having accompanied others through our attentive listening, we hope that they will not remain with the same heavy hearts, stuck in a crisis.

We want them to experience some movement within. In this action stage, therefore, we help people to think of possible options, set achievable goals, and identify what resources and strengths are available to help in the task of bringing inner peace.

Let's look briefly at a few ways of empowering others into action.

Problem solving rather than problem creating

The first thing we do in problem solving is to help take the focus off the problems themselves. By doing this we are not trying to avoid the problems. Instead, we attempt to separate the problems from the person who has the problems. This might sound unrealistic, but if we somehow separate the problem it gives us the space to stand back. When we are entangled with a problem then we cannot always focus too clearly, and we can easily feel overwhelmed. In this state of mind we do not so much solve our problems as create more of them!

Steps
1   What is my real problem?
2   What do I really want?
3   What options are open to me?
4   Am I ready to make a decision?
5   Why not give it a try?
6   Did it work?

When Mary's daughter came home ill from university and revealed her HIV status, that was indeed a problem enough. By her reaction to her daughter, Mary created a new set of problems that made communication even more difficult.

Some counselling techniques use what is called the Empty Chair as a way of looking at problems as separate from the person who has them. The pastoral counsellor asks the person to imagine an empty chair, then to put the particular problem into the chair so as to see themselves as separate:

Pastoral counsellor: Mary, I want you for a moment to put in that empty chair the fact that Patience is now HIV-positive and that this was due to the fact that she was raped. Now look at Patience without those two traumatic problems. What do you see? What were your feelings about her before this painful news? What were your hopes, dreams?

This invites Mary to recall that there was life before HIV. Perhaps not all her hopes and dreams are lost. It encourages her to get in touch with her real feelings towards her daughter. People need to be empowered by being reminded that they may have a problem, but they themselves are not problems. The first step in the action stage is to get the problem into perspective.

Goal setting

We all know from experience that a great deal of energy is used up when we have a problem because we carry it around in our head, going over the details time and again. Wishing that we never had the problem also wastes a great deal of energy. When we come to goal setting we need to help the person living with HIV/AIDS to give their attention to 'positive living'. Now that their HIV status is known, they can look to the resources and strengths that will enable them to choose life. Having a goal in itself gives us a reason to live. 'Why do I want to live?' 'What have I to live for?' These are crucial questions. Motivation is a key element in the fight against this life-destroying virus. All of us need a reason to live.

If we know why we want to live then we will search for strategies that help us live. Let us be very clear. A goal is not the same as an aim. Most of us suffer from time to time by being too vague about what we would like to do. We suffer from a 'New Year Resolution' way of thinking! Of course, a good many of these vague aims and intentions never see the light of day and certainly do not have much focus.

Goals move beyond aims in being clear and specific statements of what a person wants to put into practice in order to manage a problem situation.

Gerard Egan, *The Skilled Helper*

A goal focuses our attention on something specific and on something that is achievable. We then put structures in place that will help us work towards our goal. The important thing is that our goals are clear, realistic and evaluated. Let's look again at the story of Frank, whose partner Tom is dying. Death and bereavement are an area of special sensitivity for pastoral counsellors and it may seem at first that there could be no goal setting or action in this situation.

> *The pastoral counsellor has spent good time allowing Frank to tell the story of his relationship with Tom and explaining how he became sick. He has challenged some of Frank's self-defeating thinking and has helped Frank identify where his network of support will be when Tom dies. As time is moving on the pastoral counsellor is keen to help Frank say goodbye to Tom.*
>
> **Pastoral counsellor:** Frank, once Tom's parents arrive you may not get another chance to be alone with Tom. I'm wondering, even though Tom is semi-unconscious, what would you want to say to him before he dies?
>
> **Frank:** There's just too much … I wouldn't know where to begin …
>
> **Pastoral counsellor:** Keep it simple, Frank. Tell him something you'd like him to remember and take with him.
>
> **Frank:** I want him to know just how much I love him. That he has been an important part of my life. He's helped me accept myself.
>
> **Pastoral counsellor:** Those are important things for Tom to know. Why not say them to him now in a way that you know best? I will leave you together for a while, but call me if you need me.

When helping someone to formulate a goal it can often be helpful to get them to look at the obstacles that might somehow prevent them from achieving it. These 'hindering forces' can then be explored and weakened and ways of coping with them can be discussed. The important thing is not to dwell too long on the obstacles before turning attention to the forces that can help bring the goal to fruition. These 'facilitating forces' are the inner and outer resources that can be used to bring about a positive outcome. This stage in the process focuses the person's attention on the positive resources that may very well have been ignored because of looking too much at 'the problem'.

It is important that these resources, as well as the goal itself, come from the person living with HIV/AIDS and not the pastoral counsellor. It is they who have to live with their goal and so they have to formulate the plans of action that will work for them.

Role play

HIV/AIDS not only weakens a person's immune system, but it also takes away their energy and enthusiasm for life. They experience a loss of confidence in themselves and in life in general. An important aim of pastoral counselling is to restore not only a sense of perspective but also a renewed sense of confidence. Role play can be an important tool in helping people feel safe.

As pastoral counsellors we will often hear people say 'I just don't know what to do' or 'I don't know how I'm going to tell them'. Role play can help people try out difficult conversations, actions and attitudes in a safe environment. It feels artificial at first, but it can be a very empowering skill, as it gives the person an opportunity to experience what it feels like to be different, to work through the difficulties and stress. In fact, like the Empty Chair technique, role play can be used to explore past, present and future situations that we find overwhelming. We can address feelings and ways of thinking so as to imagine what life could be like if this problem/emotion were thought of in a new way.

Role play is an important experience for pastoral counsellors themselves and is one way we can practise and learn the skills that have been highlighted in this chapter. Several pastoral counsellors could work together in order to go through particular situations that they may encounter, and to try to emphasize one or other of the skills. We can help each other to grow in our ability to listen through constructive criticism.

> **Pastoral counsellor:** Mary, you've told me how fearful and ashamed you feel about approaching your daughter because you got angry with her when she told you of her HIV status and her rape at university. You've said that you want there to be reconciliation, but are nervous about 'getting it right', as you put it. Let's try now. Imagine that I am Patience. What's the most important thing you would want me to understand? Take a moment to think before starting. Then, after a while, we'll swop roles. I'll be you and you can feel what it's like to be Patience.

Homework/reflection

The miracles of Jesus often show that healing is not always something that happens at once. Healing is a process.

Read Luke 17:11–14

One of the important features of this healing miracle is that the lepers were healed as they walked to the priests. Healing needs time to happen.

The service that we offer people through our ministry of listening will not be finished in one conversation or counselling session. Of course, there can be occasions when one session is enough and the person feels so helped that they can manage on their own. Often, people need three or four occasions to express the full extent of the hurt they feel. Hence, towards the end of our time with them, we can give people some 'homework' or 'questions for reflection'. This gives a powerful sign to those we are listening to that we are not trying to solve their problems, give them advice or dismiss them. We are committed to them. Hence, we can suggest:

'I'm wondering if during the next few days you could reflect on the issues you have raised and consider which one is of the greatest importance to you – what might bring you relief.'

Or:

'As we've been talking, a particular passage of scripture has been coming into my mind. I'm wondering if you would like to pray with it and see how it throws light upon the things we have been talking about?'

We could even give as homework the goal that the person has come up with:

'You said that your goal would be to tell your parents that you are HIV-positive and we've explored how you could do that. I'm just wondering, are you ready to do this before we meet next time? Then we could talk about how it went.'

People need help to appreciate that as a pastoral counsellor you do not have a solution to their difficulties, but that you are willing to journey with them until they discover one for themselves.

One way to comprehend the enormity of the statistics of the AIDS epidemic is to remind ourselves that for every infected and affected person there is an accompanying human story. Telling these stories puts a human face to the anonymity of overwhelming statistics and gives voice to the numbing silence of fear, pain and death enwrapped in the shroud of stigma.

Colin Jones, Director, Church of the Province of Southern Africa, HIV and Aids Programme Christian Aid, *Women's Lives: Stories for World AIDS Day 2004*

Evaluations and endings

Setting a goal and highlighting the resources that will help facilitate it is only one step in the process. We need to help those to whom we are listening to realize that they need to come back and look again at how things went – what worked and what did not! It's not a game of win or lose, but building on strengths and utilizing weaknesses. Evaluation is necessary if we are going to maintain our healing, as it helps us to remain focused.

Evaluation can happen at the end of each session or at the beginning of the next, depending on what we are evaluating:

'Daniel, as we come to the end of our time together, I wonder if you could just think for a moment what has been helpful about this time, and how could it have been more helpful?'

'So, Daniel, I think we left off last time we met by your saying you were going to go to the doctor to enquire about antiretrovirals. How did you get on?'

We travel with another pilgrim who is HIV-affected or infected for as long as they wish us to keep them company. Yet we need to beware of creating a dependency, either from their side or ours. Through the listening process we can discern when is the right time to let this person walk alone. We need to know how to end once we realize that they can cope on their own or, rather, once we have helped them find a network of support, both internal and external.

There are just three more issues that we need to conclude with.

Confidentiality

It is a basic principle of pastoral counselling that we understand and maintain a high level of confidentiality. When people who are living with HIV/AIDS entrust their stories to us they do so on the understanding that we are not going to retell it wherever we go. Where there is no confidentiality, there can be no trust. So confidentiality is crucially important in the ministry of a pastoral counsellor.

Along with the concern about 'What will they think of me when I tell them this?' a person will also be wondering: 'Can I really trust them not to tell anyone else?' The importance of confidentiality may therefore seem to be obvious, but the issue is not as simple as we might at first think. Basic trust is essential at all times in our ministry of listening. This trust can only grow if a person is confident that their thoughts and feelings will not be communicated elsewhere. The person living with HIV/AIDS is already in a vulnerable state. As pastoral counsellors we must not violate their trust and cause more harm by spreading information inappropriately.

It is important at the very beginning of our helping relationship to explain our understanding of confidentiality. Some people may think that confidentiality is always 'absolute' (i.e. we never under any circumstances repeat what we have heard). It is of course important for us to keep information that we are told to ourselves, except where to do so would seriously threaten someone's well-being and safety. A few obvious examples are of a girl or young child who discloses they are being sexually abused, a woman who is being beaten regularly, or someone who feels suicidal. It would be wrong in these situations to allow them to go back into environments that are far from safe without providing proper care and support.

Stop and think

What might be the situations or issues that would cause you to consider that total and absolute confidentiality is unhelpful or even harmful?

We need to explore the idea of *shared* confidentiality. There will be occasions and situations where we need to share parts of a person's story with someone else in order to provide them with appropriate help. Often, people will begin their first session by saying something like: 'I hope I can trust you, you won't tell anyone about this will you?' The trap is that we say that we will not tell before we know what it is they are about to say! Our first task is to get the person's permission. If a trusting atmosphere has been created from the beginning, then the majority of people will accept a decision by the pastoral counsellor to look for further guidance and help. If we ourselves are unsure if it is right to break confidentiality we need to seek advice.

Confidentiality seems simple, but we need to be realistic. As a pastoral counsellor, trying to minister in the context of HIV/AIDS is demanding. We will be entrusted with some very painful stories and the burden of carrying them alone adds to a sense of loneliness. We are the bearers of other people's secrets. How do we cope with this? Later, we will look at the importance of support, but for now we need once again to underline the necessity of a firm spiritual life for those who accompany others in their suffering. The key to confidentiality is trust. The guideline as to how we practise confidentiality is what is the best way to support and help this person.

Support

The sensitive and emotionally demanding nature of this ministry requires each pastoral counsellor to take seriously the need to have someone with whom they can talk, without of course breaking the trust of those whose stories have been committed to them. It was suggested earlier in this manual that we could receive that support and encouragement from other pastoral counsellors within our Christian fellowship. We could come together as a group or on a one-to-one basis to review difficult cases and situations.

Professional counsellors refer to this as *supervision*, which does not mean that someone else tells us what to do, but that we talk through some of the difficulties we are meeting and problems where we feel stuck. Supervision conveys the idea of accountability. We discuss things so as to be better able to listen freely and objectively. If we are too full, how can we hope to make space for others? We can always improve our listening. A more experienced person with whom we can occasionally talk about things can help us understand what is happening in a particular listening relationship. This is another reason why we can comply with absolute confidentiality: we need the right to consult. We do so, however, without revealing the identity of the person we are speaking about.

Support, therefore, is essential to help us as pastoral counsellors so that:

* We do not absorb and carry other people's problems. We have enough of our own!
* It acts as an early warning system.
* It enables us to take care of ourselves and not to become stressed.
* It helps us to focus on our skills as listeners.
* It challenges us to develop as a listener and gives us a resource from someone more experienced than ourselves.
* It evaluates the way we minister as a pastoral counsellor so as to encourage good practice and prevent harmful behaviour.
* It provides an opportunity to look at issues surrounding our ministry of listening and demonstrates accountability.

Our support system therefore not only protects and gives us new life, but it also protects and helps the people we are listening to. Professional counsellors all work according to a code of ethics, part of which requires supervision before practising as a counsellor. In our Christian fellowship we too need guidelines to encourage a sense of responsibility, so we can give the best service to those who we seek to help.

Networking

One of the simplest ways to help others is to know what is available in your area. The problems that people living with HIV/AIDS have are varied: medical, financial, social. We can help by knowing what there is available for those living with this virus:

* Where are the counselling and testing centres and what are they like?
* What support groups exist?
* Are there NGOs or local groups that can provide home-based care?
* Is there government or other funding available for medication?
* Where can this person find spiritual support and encouragement?

Self-supervision
Take time after listening to reflect and review:
* How did I feel as I listened?
* How did I feel about the person I was listening to?
* What skills could I see myself using well?
* Where could I have improved?
* What do I want to do differently the next time we meet?

We need to know our local scene concerning HIV/AIDS, so we can refer people when they have very practical problems. Equally, we need to be aware of where we can refer people when we realize that the problem that they have is too much for us. Recognizing that you cannot assist someone is not a sign of weakness, but a clear sign of maturity. As pastoral counsellors we need to be aware of our own strengths and weaknesses. Some people have a particular skill in listening to those in bereavement, while others are stuck when having to cope with the issue of death. Some may have special sensitivity to those who have been raped, sexually abused, who are gay or whose marriage has broken down.

As a pastoral care and counselling team in a Christian fellowship, we can share our strengths so as to know to whom we can refer people when the issue in hand is too sensitive for us.

How can all this be summarized?

Perhaps the best way to summarize this chapter is to remind ourselves that we are not trying to play at being professional counsellors. Rather, we are attempting to be professional in the way we seek to help others to help themselves.

A structure does not have to make us ridged and formal; it is there to empower us to be free and spontaneous. We must above all recall the three core qualities that we bring to our helping relationship. We try by all means to enter into the world of the person who is sharing (empathy). We show the greatest respect to them as human beings through our non-judgemental attitudes (positive regard). We must be naturally ourselves in our response and compassion (genuineness).

Basic rules for counselling
- Listen with undivided attention
- Remember important details
- Relax and help others to relax
- Listen beneath the obvious
- Listen to yourself
- Listen to the still small voice within
- Avoid speaking too much
- Be sensitive in asking the right kind of questions
- Avoid judgement

Adapted from Michael Jacobs, *Still Small Voice*

As pastoral counsellors we come with the heart and compassion of God to be a channel of his healing love. We can use whatever helps us to reflect that healing presence in order to bring peace and encouragement.

Case Studies

In this chapter we will look at a variety of case studies and put into practice what we have read.

How can the church break the silence and the stigma surrounding HIV/AIDS, and take every opportunity to heal our hurting communities by being active partners in HIV/AIDS prevention, the provision of quality care, and the mitigation of its impact? We believe that the resources of the church: its scripture, its liturgy, its values, its members, its leadership and its buildings, are powerful weapons and resources for energizing and awakening the church to play its role effectively in the fight against HIV/AIDS.

Musa Dube, *Africa Praying*

The case studies in this chapter provide a wide range of possible situations for people living with HIV/AIDS. These are real life situations which you may encounter as a pastoral counsellor. How would you respond?

The purpose here is not to encourage you to build up a series of set responses. That is not possible. Each person is unique, even if their problems appear the same, and each person experiences a situation differently. The purpose of these case studies is to give you time and opportunity to reflect and to use your imagination to put yourself creatively into real situations. What are your options? What would be your main goal in helping each individual? How do you react internally to their story?

In order to help you with these case studies we ask you to imagine that they form the basis of a counselling conversation. Write out how you would guide the person through the different stages of exploring, understanding and acting. Write as if you were writing a radio play with two characters: the pastoral counsellor and the person who needs to talk. After the first case study we will provide a short example of what we mean.

> **Case study 1: Samuel**
> Samuel is a very talented young man, aged 23, strong and healthy. He plays in the youth band at church and in a jazz band at nights and weekends. For some time he has been feeling unwell. In particular he is very tired most of the time and has lost his appetite and wakes up at night in sweats. For months he has had a cough that simply will not go away. Eventually, he decides to go for a check at the local clinic and they suggest an HIV test. After some thought he has the test and he is told that he is HIV-positive. Once he is given the results he loses interest in life and tries to hide himself away. He even stops going to church. Though his friends do not know about his HIV status, they can see that something is wrong. After talking with the minister, they suggest to Samuel that he consider meeting the pastoral counsellor. When he eventually makes an appointment he comes into your room and starts to cry for a long time.

* How do you cope with tears?
* What would be your thoughts and feelings as he sat and cried?
* What would be the most helpful way you could respond?

> **A possible counselling session**
> **Pastoral counsellor:** *(After sitting in silence for a while)* Samuel, take your time ... Let the tears come ... Don't feel embarrassed for me. Just let the tears flow ...
> *(Once the tears have stopped and he seems calmer)*
> Samuel, when you feel ready, perhaps you can tell me what those tears are about.
> **Samuel:** Where do I begin, it's just all too much.
> **Pastoral counsellor:** There seems to be a great deal weighing you down, so don't try saying it all at once, but maybe help me understand what has happened that has made you want to come and talk.
> **Samuel:** I've not been well and I received bad news and kind of

went to pieces. I stopped going to church and playing in the band and I guess my friends felt I just need to talk to someone.

Pastoral counsellor: So your health has not been good and you are worried because of the bad news you received. Samuel, you seem to agree with your friends' suggestion that you needed to talk to someone, so I wonder whether it's your health or the bad news that you received that you need to talk about?

Samuel: They're linked ... OK, let me start. I wasn't well for a while. Usually, I'm fit. I work out and I am strong. Somehow I began to feel tired and run down. So eventually I went to the doctor and he suggested doing a blood test for all kinds of things ... *(Silence)*

Pastoral counsellor: *(Holds the silence for a while)* Samuel, I can see this is difficult, so take your time and then tell me what happened when you went back to get your results.

Samuel: It was then that the doctor told me ... he said ... he said I was HIV-positive. So I might as well die now! It's going to happen anyway. How can I face people? My parents would die if they knew, as for the rest ... they'd just run away from me. So that's why I shut myself away.

Pastoral counsellor: So once you heard the news of your HIV status you felt as if that was it, life had finished and I'm picking up that you were/are very concerned about what others think and how they may react to your being positive. All those are important issues which you might like to look at, Samuel, but I wonder if you were to put what other people think to one side – what's the most important thing for you at this moment?

Why not continue this conversation and practise taking Samuel through the different stages of exploring, understanding and acting on it? You cannot do everything in one conversation. Your time is limited. So by the end of this session what would your aim and goal be for Samuel? Is there anything you'd like him to reflect on before you meet again?

Another way to practise your skills is to ask a friend to help – perhaps someone else from your Christian fellowship or church who wants to be a pastoral counsellor. You could role play the case studies, taking it in turns to be the person living with HIV/AIDS and the pastoral counsellor. Discuss what it feels like to be the one counselled and sitting in the hot seat of the pastoral counsellor.

The important thing is not just to read these case studies, but to use them as a valuable source of experience. Behind these stories are real people with real life problems.

> **Case study 2: Miriam**
>
> Miriam is a successful businesswoman, well respected and admired in her place of work. Up to now she has put all her energy into developing her career with the support and encouragement of her husband, but now is the time to think of starting a family. When she suspected that she was pregnant she was very excited and went to the doctor for a check up. As part of the medical procedure it was routine for the doctor to do a blood test and a whole range of other tests, including an HIV test. After the examination Miriam was asked to return to the clinic in a week's time, when she would be given the news that confirmed her pregnancy.
>
> On the appointed day Miriam stopped off one evening from work in order to collect the results. She'd planned a special meal for her husband in order to celebrate the good news. The doctor seemed serious when she entered his room. He told Miriam that she was indeed pregnant but that her blood test had also revealed that she was HIV-positive. She was very shocked. How could this be? Had the doctor made some mistake and mixed up her results with someone else's? She couldn't be HIV-positive, as she had not had sexual relations with any other men but her husband. Nor had she been involved in any other risky behaviour. This was surely a mistake. Then slowly she began to think: 'If I am HIV-positive does that mean my husband is also positive?'
>
> She left the clinic and instead of going straight home she called in at the house of her minister. She had to talk to someone. As you invite her in you are aware that she has been crying and looks quite shocked. After a moment's silence she says:
>
> 'I don't really know how to say this, but it's as if my whole life has come to a standstill. I'm numb. I've just come from the clinic where I was to pick up my pregnancy results ... but I got more than I bargained for. I'm pregnant all right but they found out that I'm HIV-positive. How can that be? What am I to do? How do I tell Joe? You've got to help me!'

* How would you begin to help Miriam?
* What kind of opening response would you make?
* How would you reflect back what you had heard and picked up in terms of feelings?

✳ From the little she has said what issues immediately come to your mind that she might need to work through? How would you convey that to her?

✳ In what way could you assist Miriam to break the news to her husband?

✳ Would there be any value in seeing them together sometime in the future? If so, what issues are they likely to need to confront?

Case study 3: Naomi

Naomi is a widow and lives in a very poor neighbourhood with her daughter-in-law Ruth, who has three children. Naomi's only son, who had been married to Ruth, died two years ago, leaving Ruth as the only source of income. Ruth works in the evenings in a local bar as a waitress. For some months she has been feeling unwell, coughing a great deal and with constant diarrhoea. The doctor told her that she has tuberculosis and AIDS.

Naomi is very worried about how she will cope if Ruth dies. How is she to feed the children and pay their school fees? When Ruth gets too sick to work who will provide the food and medication?

Naomi sends a message to the parish house to see if Sister Rosemary would call. When you arrive you see just how poor these people are and how depressed Naomi is. 'Just tell me what am I to do … why has God done this to me now that I am old? When Ruth dies, who is going to care for us? Will God do a miracle if I pray?'

✳ Where would you begin in your response to Naomi?

✳ How would you try to explore the question of God?

✳ Where is God to be found in this pandemic?

✳ As you explore the story of Naomi's difficulties what practical resources could you offer?

✳ Do you know the possible resources in your own area where people may get help?

Case study 4: Peter

Peter is just 17 years old and the only child of the local Anglican vicar. He is bright, though recently his school work has deteriorated and his reports from school have not been good. He has developed a habit of turning up late and falling asleep in class. His parents have spoken to him about it, but he say's there's no problem. There have also been arguments about his coming home late. The relationship at home is strained.

On a day when his parents are away for a conference, Peter is rushed to hospital. At first, the doctors think it is an overdose, but it turns out that Peter has bought some bad drugs off a dealer. He also has an STI and genital warts. As the chaplain of the hospital you are asked to visit him to see if he will open up. He has told the staff that he doesn't want his parents to know. After some strained conversation he suddenly says:

'Okay, let's cut the small talk: you've been sent to find out stuff from me. I know they've told you about why I'm in here. Well, did they also tell you the latest piece of news, I'm HIV-positive? ... I wish the drugs had seen me off ... I'm in a right mess. I can see the headlines now: "Vicar's son a drug addict and has sex in the park with men to pay for them." What's my girlfriend going to do? I've probably given her this thing too. I don't know why I'm bothering to tell you this because you're probably like my dad, you've already sent me to hell.'

✳ As you listen to Peter blurt out his story what thoughts and feelings go through your mind?

✳ Now that he has stopped talking how are you going to respond?

✳ What would you like to clarify to enable the whole story of Peter's life to be told?

✳ In terms of the action stage, what might bring the most help to him in the short term and then in the long term?

Case study 5: Abel and his three wives

You are the nurse counsellor at the rural clinic. Abel and his family live near the mission station and come to the clinic when they are in need of medical attention. Over the past two months Abel's third wife, a young girl of 20, has come because she is pregnant. You know that the first wife has tested positive for HIV and that the husband has come on several occasions with STIs. You explain that it is the policy of the clinic to test pregnant women for HIV because you have a programme that tries to reduce mother to child transmission. You ask the young woman if she is willing to be tested and she agrees.

A week before she is due to return for her results the second wife comes to see you and she has a sexually transmitted disease and the beginning of herpes. You ask her if she would be willing to be tested for HIV and she refuses. When the third wife returns for her results she tells you that the first wife has died and that she herself was beaten by her husband for having an HIV test; her results are negative. 'But what if my husband is not negative? The second wife is also not too well and has a rash all over her body and a discharge from below ... My husband said only prostitutes get AIDS ... What am I to do? I don't want to die! Has my husband or the other wives come to you because they are sick? You have to tell me!'

* How would you be feeling about this family situation?
* What are the issues for you that this problem raises?
* While maintaining confidentiality how would you help the young woman protect herself?
* What are the structures in your local area and culture that might help you?

Case study 6: Zach and Elizabeth

Zach and Elizabeth have four children. Their youngest child, John, was rushed into hospital after he was knocked down by a passing car. Fortunately, the injuries were not as bad as they first thought and they were greatly relieved. Then the doctor asked to see them. He explained that as a routine procedure all blood is tested for HIV and young John was found to be positive. Both parents were shocked and on their way home they call in to see you as a friend and leader of the women's fellowship at the church they attend. You are also a pastoral counsellor. Having told you the news they blurt out:

'How could this happen to us as Christians? Why has God cursed us? We simply cannot believe that this could happen! What will happen to our family? Do we all need to go through this humiliating test? As we were driving here we thought it best to keep it a secret – can you imagine if they found out at his school? In fact, Zach and I are really wondering if the rest of the children need to know or couldn't we just keep it to ourselves and remain quiet? After all, why disturb him? With medication he may never need to know. Anyway, he won't understand. Now, please tell us what we should do!'

✳ How would you respond to the request to tell them what to do?
✳ What is the major issue that Zach and Elizabeth have not raised but is implied in their reaction to the news of their son's HIV status?
✳ If you had to list the issues mentioned in order of priority what would they be?
✳ Would you know where Zach and Elizabeth could find support in your local area?
✳ Would you find any conflict between your friendship and the relationship as a pastoral counsellor?

Case study 7: Hannah, David and Teresa

Hannah and David have three daughters. They live in an affluent area of the city and life has treated them kindly until Teresa, their second daughter, comes home one day very distressed. All at once she announces to her parents:

'I've got something terrible to tell you. My boyfriend Samuel has just told me that he's been for a second HIV-test and he's positive. I know you never wanted me to go out with him, you said he'd "been around" and wasn't good enough for a Christian girl like me. Well, what am I to do now?'

The parents call you round to help them.

✳ Where would you begin in the helping process?
✳ What information do Teresa and her parents need from you?
✳ What are the issues that have not yet been expressed but lie beneath the surface?
✳ What kind of support could you offer the family in your Christian fellowship?
✳ What help would you offer Teresa and Samuel?

Case study 8: Pastor Jeremiah

Pastor Jeremiah is a very concerned and hard working minister. He has a very kind heart and has for some time been counselling people with HIV and AIDS. His ministry also meant that he tried to care for people physically. However, he has not always been careful when dealing with bodily fluids. He has just found out that he is HIV-positive. His congregation were very unhappy about his work. He comes to see you as a fellow pastoral counsellor.

'What am I to do? How can I possibly tell the congregation? They already think I am in league with the devil, so now they will call me immoral! Then there is my wife! You have to tell me what I can do. Perhaps I should simply tell no one and get funding for antiretrovirals.'

✳ What are some of the important ethical issues that you would want to guide the pastor through?

✳ How would you begin the counselling session?

✳ To whom might you be able to refer the pastor in order to get him support?

✳ How might you help him break the news to his wife?

Case study 9: Father Pedro

You are a Catholic priest and you are asked to visit a married couple who sound distressed. Daniel, the husband, has come to you for confession over a number of years and revealed that he has occasionally had sex with men while away on business. You think that his wife, Debra, has now found out. She says:

'I really don't know how to tell you this, my life has just come to an end … I've just found out that I'm HIV-positive. I'm so angry with Daniel. He must have given it to me, as I've never had sex with anyone else. He just won't admit that he's been seeing other women while away on those business trips. Now you're here he's got to be honest.'

'Father, you've got to tell Debra the truth, I've not had sex with other women!'

✳ What thoughts and feelings are going through your mind?

✳ How would you deal with the issue of confidentiality and confession?

✳ In what ways could you help this couple come to terms with what is happening between them?

✳ What would be your main aim in this first counselling session?

✳ Who would you find to help you in this dilemma?

Using Prayer and Scripture

This chapter suggests how we can use prayer and scripture as tools in our pastoral care and counselling.

If each day a word of the Lord can truly come alive for us and can form our minds and hearts, we will come indeed to live by faith ... we will have that mind of Christ ... In this way we come to live the first great commandment to love the Lord our God with our whole mind, our whole heart, our whole soul, our whole strength.

Basil Pennington, *Seek His Mind*

HIV/AIDS is an invitation to live. As Christians who are committed to a gospel of life and hope, we must try through our pastoral care and counselling to encourage people to choose life. We can help them to cherish their God-given gift of life, despite HIV/AIDS. The HIV/AIDS pandemic is a challenge to our very survival. We must use every opportunity and every weapon we have to stay alive.

Read Ephesians 6:10–20

In this encouraging passage of scripture Paul says that we should imagine ourselves engaged in warfare and so put on all the necessary armour of God. In the fight against HIV/AIDS the weapons that Paul speaks of are very powerful:

* **Truthfulness**
* **Bring peace**
* **Justice**
* **Faith**
* **Word of God**
* **Prayer**

Paul suggests that we draw our strength from the Lord and from his mighty power. To fight in the battle against HIV/AIDS we need all the resources that we can muster. Our pastoral care must of course involve a great deal of practical assistance, but we should never forget the spiritual needs of those whom we are trying to help, nor neglect the spiritual weapons that we possess as people of faith. Among these weapons are prayer and scripture.

As pastoral counsellors who listen from the perspective of our Christian faith, we should not forget that prayer is an indispensable preparation for our ministry of listening with love. Prayer helps us to create a space within so that we can be truly available to others. During our time with those living with HIV/AIDS we can begin with prayer and use it at other appropriate times during a session. Prayer is not the last hope, but the continual support that points us to the presence of God.

The word of God is another crucial weapon in building hope and faith in the fight against a deadly virus of despair and depression. The word of God can help focus our thoughts and challenge some of our more negative and destructive ways of thinking. Reflecting on scripture can be a powerful way for those involved in pastoral counselling and those living with HIV/AIDS to look again at what gives them life.

This chapter will help you apply prayer and scripture in the fight against HIV/AIDS and enhance your apostolate of listening love. It will encourage you to add your own prayers and scripture passages to build up a living resource.

Prayers for different occasions

By a person living secretly with HIV/AIDS

My God, you know how I have struggled since I discovered I was HIV-positive! I was mad at myself and I was angry with the one who gave me this disease. Above all I was angry at you for letting this terrible thing happen to me. I am ashamed to tell anyone in case they reject me and are ashamed to know me.

Lord, I've had to learn a hard lesson. I cannot look for acceptance from others until I accept myself. This I found very difficult, but I am getting there slowly. I thank you for helping me to struggle for this acceptance. I know more than ever that you do not reject me, you are not ashamed of me, you love me.

With this strength help me now to love myself and break the deadly silence that wants to keep me a prisoner of guilt and shame. Help me to tell the people who are important to me about my status, so I can find help and support. Help me to tell them soon so as to find peace of mind.

Give me your strength so that I can now choose to live positively and choose to live fully. Amen.

For the carers

Father, your name is love. Strengthen and encourage those who have the task of caring, helping and counselling your people living with HIV and AIDS. Comfort those who try to comfort the lonely, guide those who attempt to guide those who feel lost, and give hope to us all so that we will never be overcome by despair. We ask this in the name of Jesus, our brother and healer. Amen.

Lighting a candle of hope

Lord, as I light this candle I recall your presence. May this light help me to remember all whose lives have been touched by HIV/AIDS. May it be a symbol of hope for all who are infected and affected. May it encourage us to work to bring an end to stigma, denial and new infections.

O candle, burn bright! May your flame instil within me a living sense of the love and compassion that shines through the healing presence of God. I make this prayer in Jesus' name. Amen.

A parent's prayer

God, I am so angry. I am so ashamed that my child has this disease called AIDS. I need you more than ever, for I do not know where to turn. I want to hide myself. I want to hide my child. I want to make up some story that is not true, for I do not want HIV/AIDS to be part of my family's life. Forgive me for my cowardice, my selfishness and anoint me with your grace in order to face life as it is. Be with all families who are struggling with this virus. Comfort them and help them not to be discouraged. Touch them with your healing love and bring peace. Amen.

For those who are dying

Look with love and compassion Lord upon [name] – who is soon to return home to you. You are full of mercy and no one is forgotten in your sight. Bless this child of yours who has carried in their body the HIV virus. Comfort them now in their pain, fill them with your hope and help them to experience your forgiveness. Call them now by name and receive them into your gentle arms as a loving parent. As for their relatives and friends, sustain them in their loss so that they can themselves choose life. Mary, mother of the suffering, pray for [name] to Jesus your son and wrap them with your motherly care. Amen.

For those who are bereaved

Lord Jesus, we ask you to bless those who mourn and are sad at the death of family members and friends. May they not be overwhelmed by grief, but receive the comfort and consolation that will help them each and every day. In days of loss and emptiness may they find in their hearts a sense of trust and hope in you, for you have broken the barrier of death and promise us life everlasting. Amen.

Litany of Hope and Compassion

Leader: Father, we know you will always hear our prayers.
People: We turn to you in all our need.
Leader: We pray for all who share in this HIV/AIDS pandemic.
People: Help us to see that in sharing in the pain of others we can grow in hope and compassion.
Leader: We prayer for all who are as yet not infected.
People: Encourage them to make wise choices so as to always choose life.
Leader: We pray for those who already carry this virus in their bodies.
People: Give them the resolve to live positively and not to lose hope.
Leader: We hold in your loving heart those who care for others in their sickness.
People: Give them patience and strength when things are hard.
Leader: We pray for the dying.
People: Welcome them home into your loving embrace.
Leader: We pray for the dead and those who mourn.
People: Bring peace to both and an experience of your eternal compassion.
All: Lord, we bring all these prayers to you in the name of your son Jesus, who is the resurrection and the life, and in the power of your Spirit who heals and makes us holy. Amen.

A child's prayer

God, if you are there, please listen.

I don't know what to say to someone so big, but I'm so confused. Why did my parents have to die? Why am I left alone? I cry myself to sleep and I don't know if I really want to live. Could you not let me die and then the pain inside would go. I'm tired of being called an orphan! I want some place to call my own. A family, a house, a life that is normal. I want love, not just kindness and charity.

So God, I'm looking to you, for you alone can give me the love I need. I have to live, so give me hope.

I can say no more. You know anyway what's inside. Just be with me now as I go to sleep. Help me get through another day. Amen.

A rosary of life and hope

First mystery: Mary conceives the Word

Mary received the angel's message, but I do not know if I can accept my status. When I received the news I was HIV-positive I felt sick at heart. Lord, give me an accepting heart. Help me to find your Word of life.

Second mystery: Mary gives birth to Jesus

When I was born a new life came into the world. Where can I find life now with this virus? Lord, I feel as if my life has come to an end, but you are born in me each time I say 'yes' to hope and life.

Third mystery: Mary names Jesus

There is pain in my body, but the deeper pain is in my spirit. I fear other people's reaction and rejection of me. What do they think of me? Lord, help me to cope with the many infections I encounter, especially the infection of stigma. Help me to call things by their proper name.

Fourth mystery: The wise men look for Jesus

Lord, I want to live, but I know that one day I will die. I fear death as I fear the pain. Teach me to find in you the mercy and compassion that I do not find in others.

Fifth mystery: The resurrection

Looking at your risen body makes me long for a day when I do not have to carry this virus around. By your death you have destroyed death. Give me courage to believe that life is victorious and hope will win out.

Some useful texts for HIV/AIDS ministry

The word of God is truly live and active. It is a word of life. If we are to help those living with HIV/AIDS to live positively we need to help them discover the truth that can set them fee. Often, we hear that proper nutrition is crucial for living with this virus. The nutrition we need is not only for our physical bodies, but also our minds and hearts. Reading scripture can really be a gift that frees us from negative thoughts and feelings that take away our energy. So let's add God's word to our daily diet.

Take your Bible into your hands and remember it contains the living word of God. As Dietrich Bonhoeffer said: 'The heart of God opens itself up to us in God's word.' Ask the Holy Spirit to help you to read this sacred text. As we invite the Holy Spirit to help us to listen, we open ourselves to receive a word that will help us live through the day.

We then read slowly and listen to the passage before us. We may read through the passage several times, so that it sinks deep within us. How does it speak to our situation? How can I apply its healing ointment to the wounds that I carry?

We then choose a word or phrase that we will take into our daily living and continue to pray with it.

This is a simply way to be with God's word of life and to allow it to empower us. Below, we will find a selection of Bible passages. We can add more as we find time each day to sit with God's healing word.

Genesis 1 and 2	Creation story	Created in the image and likeness of God / Human dignity and destiny
Genesis 28:10–16	Jacob's dream	We struggle to find God in the context of HIV/AIDS, but God reminds us we are standing on Holy ground / He is present. What is our dream?
Ezekiel 36:1–14	Dry bones	Choice in life / New life / Resurrection
Ezekiel 47:1–12	Vision of water	Invitation to enter the depths and find healing
Deuteronomy 30:11–end	Moses invites choice	Choice of life rather than death – living positively
1 Kings 19:9–13	Elijah's experience of God	Prayer of stillness: where is God's voice in this virus?
1 Samuel 3:1–9	Call of Samuel	Listening to God's call
Psalm 23	Shepherd	Direction / Being led
Psalm 27	Confidence in God	Seeking God / Hope
Psalm 40	I waited for the Lord	Patience / Reassurance
Psalm 42	Yearning for God	Prayer
Psalm 62	You are my God	Longing
Psalm 85	God of promise	Invitation to find hope
Psalm 103	Bless the Lord	Healing / Forgiveness
Mark 2:15–17	Jesus eats with sinners	Breaking stigma and discrimination
Mark 5:1–20	Demoniac	Being set free from stigma and discrimination / Responsibility
Mark 5:25–34	Woman of faith	Invitation to faith / Role of women in HIV/AIDS context / Gender issues / What are you looking for?

Mark 6:45–52	Walking on the water	Courage / Faith / Trust / Storms of life
Matthew 5:13–16	We are the light of the world	We must let our light shine out for others in hope
Matthew 13:24–30	Weeds and wheat	Strength and weakness / Self-acceptance
Matthew 25:31–46	Sheep and goats	We will be judged by the quality of our love
Luke 1	Annunciation / Visitation	Faith of Mary / Surrender / How has God visited you? Your Magnificat / Vocation of women in the context of HIV/AIDS
Luke 7:36–50	Washing Jesus' feet	Reconciliation / Forgiveness / Practical care
Luke 10:38–11:13	Mary and Martha	Teaching on prayer / Importance of finding time to sit at the feet of Jesus / Lord's Prayer, etc.
Luke 11:25–37	Who is your neighbour?	Who am I called to serve? / Whose wounds do I bind up and heal?
Luke 15	The prodigal son	God is all mercy / Who do you need to forgive?
Luke 18:35–45	Blind man cured	What are you asking of Jesus if you are living with HIV/AIDS? Where is your blindness?
Luke 19:1–10	Zacchaeus	Salvation comes to your house; we have a real dignity that Jesus wants to share
Luke 24:13–35	Emmaus	Jesus joins us on our journey with HIV/AIDS. He wants to listen to us. What have you learnt on your journey?
Luke 24:36–49	Appearance of Jesus	Given power / Called to witness to others and through our disclosure give hope
John 4	Samaritan woman	Jesus wants to hear the story of your life; our story can help us and give them courage
John 5:1–9	Pool of Bethesda	Do you want to be healed? What ways could you help yourself to receive healing?
John 9	Man born blind	What/where is your blindness? Stigma and discrimination
John 10	Good shepherd	Which voices do you listen to? How can you learn how to listen to the voice of life?
John 13	Jesus washes the disciples' feet	We are called to wash each other's feet even when we ourselves are infected
John 14	Many mansions	Jesus comes into your fears

John 15	Vine	Union with God
John 16	The Spirit	Where is the Spirit in your life?
John 20:19–29	Upper room	Jesus comes into your wounds
1 Corinthians 2	The hidden wisdom of God	Entering the mind of Christ
1 Corinthians 3:1–16	Co-workers with God	Temple of the Spirit / Even though our bodies are infected with HIV we are temples of God
1 Corinthians 12	Spiritual gifts	Where are your gifts? Look for the resources that help you live positively
1 Corinthians 13	Hymn to love	Where does my love stop?
2 Corinthians 1:3–11	Blessed be God	Our suffering has a purpose
2 Corinthians 3:7–18	The veil of Moses	Called to transformation
2 Corinthians 4:5–15	Treasure in clay	We carry Jesus within our HIV/AIDS infected bodies
2 Corinthians 5:14–21	Message of reconciliation	We are in Christ and held in love. Who do we need to forgive?
Romans 6	Baptism	We have died and risen in Christ
Romans 8:1–17	Life through the Spirit	Our dignity as children of God
Romans 8:18–27	Filled with the Spirit	God comes in our weakness
Romans 8:28–39	Not separate from God	Held in love
Galatians 5:16–25	Fruit of the Spirit	Where is your fruit?
Ephesians 1:3–14	Blessed be God	We are blessed even though we are infected or affected
Ephesians 2:4–10	Rich in mercy	Importance of mercy and grace
Ephesians 3:14–21	Paul's prayer	Self-knowledge
Ephesians 4	Become perfect	Vocation and challenge
Ephesians 6:10–20	Armour of God	Self-help in the spiritual life
Philippians 2:1–11	Hymn to Christ	Being Christ-like; humility
Philippians 3:7–16	To know Christ	Call to maturity
Colossians 1:10–14	Lifestyle	Life in Christ
Colossians 1:15–21	Christ, image of God	Bearers of God's image
Colossians 3:1–9	Seek the things of heaven	Where is your vision?
Colossians 3:10–17	Put on the new self	Call to change
James 3	The tongue	Invitation to truth
1 John 1	Walk in the light	Choose life
1 John 3:1–6	The love of the Father	Bathe in God's love
Revelation 21:1–7	A new heaven	Called to be with God
Revelation 22:1–5	River of life	Where is the river of life for you?

Glossary

We have tried not to use too many technical words, but in your work as a pastoral counsellor you will find the following material of great use.

accountability As a means of safeguarding ourselves and the persons we seek to help, pastoral counsellors should work within a recognized code of ethics and good practice. Codes of conduct can be obtained from:
BC&P, 1 Regent Place, Rugby CV21 2PJ, United Kingdom.
Association of Christian Counsellors, 173a Workington Road, Reading, RG6 1LT, United Kingdom.
Methodist Publishing House, 20 Ivatt Way, Peterborough, PE3 7PG, United Kingdom.

active listening The skill of giving the person we are listening to our full and undivided attention.

affected persons Those who find themselves associated with those living with HIV/AIDS.

AIDS Acquired Immune Deficiency Syndrome. It is caused by a virus, which impairs the body's ability to fight infection, making the body especially susceptible to frequent and random infections. These are known as opportunistic infections. The most common among them include pneumonia, tuberculosis and certain cancers such as Kaposi's sarcoma, which affects the skin.

antiretrovirals (ARVs) Drugs that reduce the levels of HIV in the bloodstream.

CD4 receptors Also known as T-helper cells. One can imagine them as officers in the body's army of defence which protect you against infection and disease.

challenge/confrontation A skill that invites the pastoral counsellor to bring to the attention of a person any inconsistencies and inaccurate information they may have.

Christian listening There are Christians who have understood the importance of listening as a way of healing and growth. They are willing to make contact with those infected by HIV/AIDS, the bereaved, long-term carers and those struggling with the virus. They are willing to visit people in their homes, hospitals, refugee camps and prisons in order to offer pastoral care, counselling and support.

community of faith The local church or Christian fellowship to which a person belongs or to which a pastoral counsellor is attached.

confidentiality An agreed commitment not to speak about what has been discussed in counselling except when someone's safety and well-being are in great danger.

empathy The ability to enter into the experience and feelings of another person as if they were one's own. We see things from the perspective of the other person so as to gain emotional understanding.

genuineness The ability to be oneself; to be real, honest and sincere. An important quality for those who wish to be pastoral counsellors.

HIV Human Immunodeficiency Virus, which can eventually cause AIDS. People infected with HIV may look and feel well for a number of years before any opportunistic infections develop. Many people infected with the HIV virus are completely unaware of the fact, unless they decide to have a blood test. However, they can be carriers of the virus, transmitting it to others.

HIV test A laboratory test made on a small sample of blood, which detects whether HIV antibodies are present in the blood. Though the presence of antibodies indicates that the person has been exposed to the virus, their absence does not necessarily mean that the person is not infected with HIV. Once we are infected we can pass on the HIV virus even though it may not yet have been found in our blood. The HIV test does not indicate that a person will go on to develop full-blown AIDS.

HIV-positive Indicates that HIV antibodies are present in the blood of the person tested. If the test is positive it means that the person has been exposed to HIV infection and that their immune system has developed antibodies to the virus.

immune deficiency The impairment of the body's ability to resist infection.

immune system The body's natural defence system, which protects it from infection by recognizing bacteria, viruses and disease in general. It consists of cells that among other things produce antibodies, which recognize materials as foreign to the body and then attempt to neutralize them without injury to other cells.

infected persons Persons who have been tested for HIV and found to be positive. They have the virus within their bodies.

opportunistic infections An infection caused by an otherwise harmless micro-organism that can become pathogenic (i.e. cause or produce disease) when the host's resistance is impaired.

pastoral counselling There are many definitions of counselling. The one chosen here highlights the pastoral context of the activity in the light of HIV/AIDS. Pastoral counselling is a helping relationship undertaken by women and men of faith in which one person agrees explicitly to give time, attention and respect to another person infected or affected by HIV/AIDS so that they have an opportunity to explore the thoughts, feelings and behaviour that their present situation brings about. Pastoral counselling recognizes the particular importance of questions of faith as well as ultimate concerns about life and death, values and meanings. Its aim is to help people to discover and clarify ways of living more resourcefully and to enable them to achieve a greater sense of well-being. It is a relationship with a purpose that is carried out within agreed boundaries in which one person helps others to help themselves.

pastoral counsellor A Christian who sees the importance of a 'ministry of listening' and having undergone some basic training in counselling skills is willing to give people living with HIV/AIDS, as well as members of their families and those most affected, time and opportunity within a formal or informal setting to explore the issues that deeply trouble them.

person infected/affected A term used to denote an individual seeking pastoral counselling. It has been chosen in preference to many other possibilities, such as 'recipient', 'church member' or 'client'. 'Person' is used to show that each individual has the right to be treated with dignity, respect and sensitivity as an equal child of God. Someone infected or affected with HIV/AIDS is first and foremost a person, not a problem or disease.

References and Further Reading

Bailey, Anne (1996), *One New Humanity*, SPCK: London.

Bate, Stuart C. (ed.) (2003), *Responsibility in a Time of AIDS*, Cluster Publications: Pietermaritzburg.

Cassidy, Sheila (1991), *Good Friday People*, Darton, Longman and Todd: London.

Christian Aid (2004), *Women's Lives: Stories for World AIDS Day 2004*, Christian Aid: London.

Dube, Musa (2003), *Africa Praying*, World Council of Churches: Geneva.

Dube, Musa (2003), *HIV/AIDS and the Curriculum: Methods of Integrating HIV/AIDS in Theological Programmes*, World Council of Churches: Geneva.

Egan, Gerard (1990), *The Skilled Helper*, Brooks/Cole: Florence, KY.

Frankl, Victor (2004), *Man's Search for Meaning*, Rider: New York.

Guenther, Margaret (1992), *Holy Listening*, Cowley Publications: Cambridge, MA.

Institute of Counselling (2000), *Introduction to Counselling*, Institute of Counselling: Glasgow.

Jacobs, Michael (1982), *Still Small Voice: An Introduction to Pastoral Counselling*, SPCK: London.

Long, Ann (1990), *Listening*, Darton, Longman and Todd: London.

Muchiri, John (1999), *HIV/AIDS: Breaking the Silence*, Nairobi: Pauline Publications Africa.

Neen, Michael and Dryden, Windy (2002), *Life Coaching: A Cognitive-Behavioural Approach*, Brunner-Routledge: London.

Nelson-Jones, Richard (1997), *Practical Counselling and Helping Skills*, Cassel: London.

Nouwen, Henri (1976), *Reaching Out*, Collins: London.

O'Donohue, M. and Vitillo, R J. (1997), *CARITAS Training Manual on the Pandemic HIV/AIDS*, Nairobi: Pauline Publications Africa.

Parry, Sue (2003), *Response of the Faith-Based Organizations to HIV/AIDS in Sub-Saharan Africa*. World Council of Churches: Geneva.

Pennington, Basil (2002), *Seek His Mind*, Paraclete Press.

Rogers, Carl (2003), *On Becoming A Person*, Mariner Books: Boston, MA.

Slattery H. (2002), *HIV/AIDS – A Call to Action: Responding as Christians*, Nairobi: Pauline Publications Africa.

Smith, Ann and McDonagh, Enda (2003), *The Reality of HIV/AIDS*, Trocare/Veritas/Cafod.

UNAIDS (2004), *2004 Report on the Global AIDS Epidemic*. United Nations: New York.

WCC (1997), *Facing AIDS: The Challenge, the Churches' Response*, World Council of Churches: Geneva.

WCC (2001), *Plan of Action*, World Council of Churches: Geneva.

WCC (2003), *Africa Praying: A Handbook on HIV/AIDS Sensitive Sermon Guidelines and Liturgy*, World Council of Churches: Geneva.

Weinreich, Sonja and Benn, Christoph (2004), *AIDS: Meeting the Challenge*, World Council of Churches: Geneva.

Whiteside, Alan and Sunter, Clem (2000), *AIDS: The Challenge for South Africa*, Human Rousseau Tafelberg: Stellenbosch.

Williams, G. and Williams, A. (eds.) (2002), *Journeys of Faith*, TALC.

Imprimé en France par I.M.E.
25110 Baume-les-Dames
Dépôt légal : août 2005